MRCS Picture Questions

Book 2

Edited by

Tjun Tang MRCS
*Clinical Research Associate
and Honorary Specialist Registrar (Vascular Surgery)
Cambridge University Hospital NHS Foundation Trust*

and

BV Praveen MS FRCS (Ed) FRCS (Eng) FRCS (Glasg) FRCS (Ire) FRCS (Gen)
*Consultant Surgeon
Southend University Hospital
Honorary Clinical Senior Lecturer
Queen Mary University of London
and Examiner, Intercollegiate MRCS Examination*

Foreword by

Pradip K Datta MS FRCS (Ed) FRCS (Eng) FRCS (Glasg) FRCS (Ire)
*Honorary Secretary of RCS (Ed)
and Examiner MRCS Examinations*

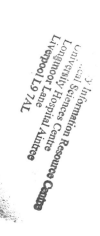
Radcliffe Publishing
Oxford • Seattle

Radcliffe Publishing Ltd
18 Marcham Road
Abingdon
Oxon OX14 1AA
United Kingdom

www.radcliffe-oxford.com
Electronic catalogue and worldwide online ordering facility.

New research and clinical experience can result in changes in treatment and drug therapy. Readers of this book should therefore check the most recent product information on any drug they may prescribe to ensure they are complying with the manufacturer's recommendations concerning dosage, the method and duration of administration, and contraindications. Neither the publisher nor the authors accept liability for any injury or damage arising from this publication.

British Library Cataloguing in Publication Data

A catalogue record for this book is available from the British Library.

ISBN-10: 1 84619 054 1
ISBN-13: 978 1 84619 054 4

Typeset by Advance Typesetting Ltd, Oxfordshire.
Printed and bound by Alden Press (Malaysia).

Contents

Foreword

It gives me great pleasure to write a foreword to this book, not least because I have known Mr Praveen ever since his pre-Fellowship days shortly after he came to the UK in the early 1990s. Now, as a Consultant Surgeon in Southend, he has established himself as a good, enthusiastic and committed surgical teacher.

In this day and age surgical teachers are a rare breed. If one was to 'triage' the responsibilities of a surgeon in the NHS, teaching would end up pretty low in the order of priorities – first comes service provision (and quite rightly too), then 'number-crunching' of patients treated to keep managers happy, private practice, research and family. Praveen has been able to strike a superb balance with considerable emphasis on teaching. This book is the outcome of the painstaking collection of clinical material over many years by the two editors, aided by colleagues who have contributed much towards this very worthwhile publication.

Surgical trainees sometimes go from pillar to post in search of good teaching. The MRCS trainees should consider themselves lucky to have this book to prepare for the examination. As an examiner for the MRCS, I can assure the reader that this book comprehensively covers every aspect of Surgery in General including pathology, and answers all questions that can conceivably be asked either in the MCQs or Final Assessment. Some of the material is in such detail that I dare say the book would also be useful for the Higher Surgical Trainee preparing for the Exit FRCS examination.

As a person in the autumn of his surgical career, it gives me immense personal pleasure to see this publication come to fruition – edited by two very committed young teachers, ably supported by several consultants and up and coming young surgeons who are setting out on the road to a surgical vocation. 'A picture is equal to a thousand words' – this adage is exemplified by the excellent pictures in this volume generously contributed by many young surgeons.

In writing this foreword, I must be careful not to stray into making it a 'book review'; that must be somebody else's job. All I can say is that the reader will find the following pages a compelling read. The quality of authorship is such that I will be surprised if other books did not soon emerge from the same stable. I wish the two authors every success.

Pradip K Datta
MS FRCS (Ed), FRCS (Eng),
FRCS (Ire), FRCS (Glasg)
Honorary Secretary and College Tutor
The Royal College of Surgeons of Edinburgh
Honorary Consultant Surgeon, Caithness
General Hospital, Wick
October 2006

Preface

It gives us great pleasure to present our book to you. It is designed for candidates sitting both the new intercollegiate MRCS examination as well as the undergraduate clinical examinations in surgery. The method of presentation and topics are drawn from our own experiences during preparation for our examinations. The book provides visual revision material to reinforce core subject matter. The questions are based around a photograph or a set of pictures with each question slightly more difficult than the previous one.

With the new European Working Time Directive and the reduction in doctors' hours, trainees may find it more difficult to be exposed to all the different clinical cases. The MRCS examination requires candidates to acquire knowledge of the presentation and appearance of a wide range of surgical problems and we believe this book allows students and trainees to acquire useful packages of information, not only for examination purposes but also to help them during their clinical practice. The combination of clinical photos and questions is perhaps the best way to revise both the clinical aspects and the subject matter associated with them. It is also believed that seeing clinical cases and reading about them at the same time reinforces knowledge retention.

Case selection is based principally not only upon the editors' experiences but also those of other distinguished clinicians in different sub-specialties. All contributors have been through the rigours of the MRCS examination and several are current intercollegiate MRCS examiners. Typical examination subject material and questions are presented.

We hope you enjoy working your way through this picture book and please do let us have your valued comments. We wish you all the best in your examinations and surgical career.

TT
BVP
October 2006

'The conditions necessary for the surgeon are four: first, he should be learned; second, he should be expert; third, he must be ingenious; and fourth, he should learn to adapt himself.'

Guy de Chauliac, 1300–68

List of contributors

Iain Au-Yong
Specialist Registrar (Radiology)
Nottingham Rotation

Pieter Bothma
Consultant Anaesthetist and Intensivist
James Paget NHS Trust Hospital, Great Yarmouth

Christopher Constant
Consultant Orthopaedic Surgeon
Addenbrooke's NHS Trust Hospital, Cambridge

Gerald David
Clinical Fellow (General Surgery)
James Paget NHS Trust Hospital, Great Yarmouth

Bimbi Fernando
Consultant Hepatobiliary and Transplant Surgeon
Royal Free University Teaching Hospital, London

Stephen Hanna
Specialist Registrar (Neurosurgery)
Northern Deanery

Aslam Khan
Clinical Fellow (General Surgery)
James Paget NHS Trust Hospital, Great Yarmouth

Vamsi Velchuru
Clinical Fellow (General Surgery)
James Paget NHS Trust Hospital, Great Yarmouth

Acknowledgements

Vanda Amanat
Specialist Breast Nurse
James Paget NHS Trust Hospital, Great Yarmouth

Ashley Brown
Clinical Tutor and Consultant Surgeon
Southend NHS Trust Hospital, Essex

Department of Radiology
Southend NHS Trust Hospital, Essex

Jonathan Gillard
Honorary Consultant Neuroradiologist and Reader
Addenbrooke's NHS Trust Hospital, Cambridge

Roger Kittle
Medical Illustration Department
Southend NHS Trust Hospital, Essex

John Latham
Consultant Radiologist
James Paget NHS Trust Hospital, Great Yarmouth

Medical Photography Services
James Paget NHS Trust Hospital, Great Yarmouth

Saman Perera
Consultant Radiologist
Southend NHS Trust Hospital, Essex

Bruce Smith
Consultant Radiologist
James Paget NHS Trust Hospital, Great Yarmouth

Alphonse Tadross
Associate Specialist (General Surgery)
James Paget NHS Trust Hospital, Great Yarmouth

Geoffrey Waters
Consultant Histopathologist
Medical Photographer
James Paget NHS Trust Hospital, Great Yarmouth

Abbreviations

AAA	abdominal aortic aneurysm
AC	acromioclavicular
ACE	angiotensin-converting enzyme
ACS	abdominal compartment syndrome
ACTH	adrenocorticotrophic hormone
AFP	alpha-fetoprotein
AIP	acute intermittent porphyria
AJCC	American Joint Committee on Cancer
ALA	amino-laevulinic acid
ALT	alkaline transferase
AP	anterior–posterior
APD	automated peritoneal dialysis
ARDS	acute respiratory distress syndrome
AST	aspartate transaminase
ATLS	Advanced Trauma Life Support
AV	arteriovenous
AVN	avascular necrosis
AXR	abdominal X-ray
BCS	breast conservation surgery
BP	blood pressure
CAPD	continuous ambulatory peritoneal dialysis
CCPD	continuous cycling peritoneal dialysis
CDC	complement-dependent cytotoxicity
CMV	cytomegalovirus
CO	cardiac output
COPD	chronic obstructive airways disease
CPAP	continuous positive airway pressure
CPR	cardiopulmonary resuscitation
CRH	corticotrophin-releasing hormone
CRP	C-reactive protein
CSF	cerebrospinal fluid
CT	computerised tomography
CVP	central venous pressure
CXR	chest X-ray
DA	duodenal atresia
DCIS	ductal carcinoma *in situ*
DDH	developmental dysplasia of the hip
DHS	dynamic hip screw
DIEP	deep inferior epigastric perforator
DIP	distal interphalangeal
DMSA	dimercaptosuccinic acid

DSA	digital subtraction angiogram
DVT	deep vein thrombosis
EBV	Epstein–Barr virus
EC	extracapsular
ECMO	extracorporeal membrane oxygenation
ENT	ear, nose and throat
ERCP	endoscopic retrograde cholangiopancreatography
ESR	erythrocyte sedimentation rate
ETT	endotracheal tube
FBC	full blood count
FCR	flexor carpi radialis
FCU	flexor carpi ulnaris
FDP	flexor digitorum profundus
FDS	flexor digitorum superficialis
FIo_2	fraction of inspired oxygen
FNA	fine needle aspiration
FPL	flexor pollicis longus
GCS	Glasgow Coma Score
GFR	glomerular filtration rate
GH	growth hormone
GI	gastrointestinal
HCP	hereditary coproporphyria
HLA	human leucocyte antigen
IAH	intra-abdominal hypertension
IAP	intra-abdominal pressure
IC	intracapsular
ICD	intercostal drain
IGAP	inferior gluteal artery perforator
IgG	immunoglobulin G
IL-2	interleukin-2
IMHS	intramedullary hip screw
IP	interphalangeal
iv	intravenous
IVP	intravenous pyelogram
IVU	intravenous urography
LCIS	lobular carcinoma *in situ*
LD	latissimus dorsi
LFT	liver function tests
MAGPI	meatal advancement and glanuloplasty
MAST	military anti-shock trouser
MEN	multiple endocrine neoplasia
MHC	major histocompatibility complex
MI	myocardial infarction
MIBG	meta-iodobenzylguanidine
MODS	multi-organ dysfunction syndrome
MRA	magnetic resonance angiogram
MRCP	magnetic resonance cholangiopancreatogram
MRI	magnetic resonance imaging
MTP	metatarsophalangeal
NPI	Nottingham Prognostic Index
NSAID	non-steroidal anti-inflammatory drug
Pao_2	partial pressure of arterial carbon dioxide
Pao_2	partial pressure of arterial oxygen

PBG	porphobilinogen
PCWP	pulmonary capillary wedge pressure
PD	peritoneal dialysis
PEEP	positive end-expiratory pressure
PIPJ	proximal interphalangeal joint
PTC	percutaneous transhepatic cholangiography
PTFE	polytetrafluoroethylene
PTH	parathormone
RIA	radioimmunoassay
RR	relative risk
RR	respiration rate
SGAP	superior gluteal artery perforator
SIRS	systemic inflammatory response syndrome
SV	stroke volume
SVC	superior vena cava
TDC	tunnelled dialysis catheter
TIPSS	transjugular intrahepatic portosystemic shunt
TNF-α	Tumour necrosis factor-α
tPA	tissue plasminogen activator
TRAM	transverse rectus abdominis myocutaneous (flap)
U&E	urea and electrolytes
UICC	Union Internationale Contre le Cancer
USS	ultrasound scan
VMA	vanillyl mandelic acid
VP	variegate porphyria
VR	venous return

Dedicated to ...

My parents-in-law ... for their untiring service to healthcare.

Section 1

Orthopaedics

Fracture dislocation of the shoulder (1)

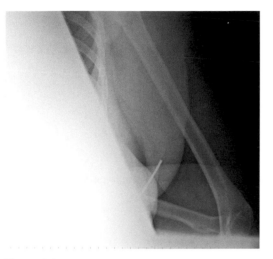

Figure 1.1

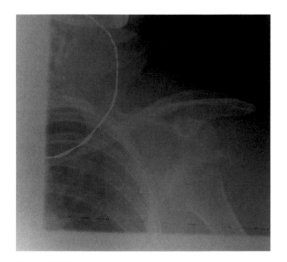

Figure 1.2

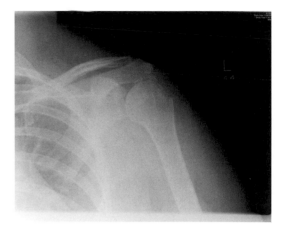

Figure 1.3

A 45-year-old female patient fell on to her outstretched hand, suffering an injury to her shoulder. These X-rays were taken on her attendance at the accident and emergency department.

Questions

Q1 Describe the injury shown on X-ray.

Q2 Discuss the management of this injury.

Q3 List the complications of this injury and the management of one of the complications.

Q4 What is the likely outcome after such an injury in a patient in her mid-40s?

Answers

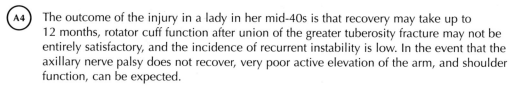

A1 The injury is a fracture dislocation of the shoulder. The dislocation is likely to be anterior, but cannot be categorically stated on a single view.

A2 Management is reduction of the fracture dislocation by any of the standard methods described.

A3 Complications are:

1 failure to reduce the fracture fragment such that it remains in the subacromial space or significantly displaced (Figure 1.3)
2 an axillary nerve palsy, or brachial plexus lesion
3 a vascular injury.

Treatments of each of these are:

1 accurate anatomical reduction of the greater tuberosity; this may require surgery and fixation
2 the axillary nerve injury may need exploration and repair
3 angiography and vascular repair.

A4 The outcome of the injury in a lady in her mid-40s is that recovery may take up to 12 months, rotator cuff function after union of the greater tuberosity fracture may not be entirely satisfactory, and the incidence of recurrent instability is low. In the event that the axillary nerve palsy does not recover, very poor active elevation of the arm, and shoulder function, can be expected.

Acromioclavicular joint osteoarthrosis

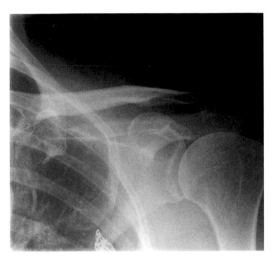

Figure 1.4

A 60-year-old patient presented with pain in the shoulder affecting primarily overhead activity, and pain on lying on the left side at night which interfered with sleep. X-rays are as shown.

Questions

Q1 What radiological diagnosis is present on this X-ray which would account for the patient's symptoms?

Q2 In the presence of reduced shoulder strength, what investigations would be appropriate, and why?

Q3 Describe the treatment of:
- osteoarthrosis of the AC joint
- subacromial impingement
- rotator cuff tear.

Answers

(A1) The radiological diagnosis is osteoarthrosis of the AC joint and irregularity of the undersurface of the acromion, a normal glenohumeral joint and slight narrowing of the subacromial space.

(A2) Further investigations would be an ultrasound to determine the integrity of the cuff, and/or an MRI scan to detect the presence of a rotator cuff tear, particularly if there is loss of strength.

(A3) Treatment of AC joint arthrosis is arthroscopic or open excision of the acromioclavicular joint; treatment of subacromial impingement is acromioplasty (either open or arthroscopic); and treatment of a rotator cuff tear is by arthroscopic or open means, if it is symptomatic – namely if there is shoulder weakness. Conservative treatment in the event that the rotator cuff tear is asymptomatic is to be recommended. Other forms of treatment include conservative treatment with anti-inflammatories and analgesics, physiotherapy, local steroid and local anaesthetic injection into the AC joint and subacromial space.

Ankle fracture

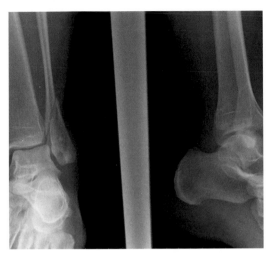

Figure 1.5

A male patient aged 30 years suffered a twisting injury to his right ankle in a football match, and was unable to weight-bear thereafter. X-rays of the right ankle are shown in Figure 1.5.

Questions

Q1 Describe the appearances of the X-ray indicating the nature of any bony or ligamentous injury that is apparent.

Q2 Name two ankle fracture classifications that you know of, and describe one in detail.

Q3 What treatment options are available to a patient with this injury?

Answers

 There is a spiral fracture of the distal fibular shaft at the level of the ankle joint, without significant displacement. There is slight lateral displacement of the talus on the tibia, opening up the medial side of the ankle, and suggesting a stretch or tear of the medial collateral ligament of the ankle.

 The two classifications that you should know are:
- *the Lauge–Hansen classification*: this classification was designed by exerting forces across the cadaveric ankle in different ways, thereby producing fractures and ligamentous injuries in sequence. Injuries are classified as supination (S), supination/external rotation (SE) or pronation (P) with or without rotation. The advantage of this classification is that the bony injuries correlate with the specific ligamentous injuries identified in the classification. This particular fracture is a supination external rotation fracture type II (SE2) in which there is a spiral fracture of the distal fibula at the level of the ankle joint in association with either a chip fracture off the tip of the medial malleolus, or in this case, distraction of the medial side of the joint indicative of a medial ligament injury.
- *the Weber classification*: this classification is based on A, B, C grading, depending on the position of the fibular fracture. Classification A is where the fibular fracture is distal to the level of the ankle joint; B is at the level of the ankle joint; and C is proximal to the level of the ankle joint. Once again this indicates the nature of the injury. This fracture would be classified as a Weber B with some lateral displacement.

 The first treatment option is conservative manipulative reduction. If the gap on the inner side of the ankle closes to normal dimensions, and the fibula remains reduced, then a conservative treatment with plaster can be recommended, with non-weight-bearing for approximately four weeks, followed by plaster cast weight-bearing for a further two to three weeks, and rehabilitation thereafter. The alternative is operative treatment, with a fibular plate, and exploration of the medial side if reduction of the medial side does not occur during surgery. Many would recommend exploration of the medial side to repair the ligament at the same time as plating, regardless of whether the reduction was complete or not. Because of the ligamentous injury, plaster casting would be recommended following surgery for a period of four to six weeks.

Bilateral total hip replacement

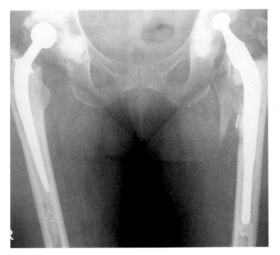

Figure 1.6

Questions

Q1 Describe the accompanying X-ray of the pelvis and hips.

Q2 Describe the complications that are visible on the left hip.

Answers

A1 This is a pelvis with bilateral proximal femur and hips. There are bilateral hip replacements present. On the right-hand side, the hip is cemented and the marker of a cement restrictor is seen distal to the prosthetic hip.

A2 On the left-hand side, the appearance is of an un-united greater tuberosity osteotomy or fracture, a periprosthetic fracture affecting the proximal shaft and lesser trochanter. A number of loose fragments of wire are visible.

Colles' fracture

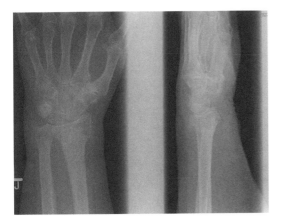

Figure 1.7

The X-ray in Figure 1.7 shows a left Colles' fracture.

Questions

Q1 Define a Colles' fracture.

Q2 After whom is it named?

Q3 What is the treatment for this fracture?

Q4 List three important complications of this fracture and describe the treatment of one of them.

Answers

(A1) A Colles' fracture is a non-articular fracture of the distal end of the radius with dorsal displacement, dorsal tilt, radial deviation and impaction, and an associated fracture of the ulnar styloid.

(A2) The fracture is named after Abraham Colles, from Dublin.

(A3) Treatment is disimpaction, correction of deformity and placement in a below-elbow cast in ulnar deviation, and wrist flexion for a period of six weeks. An above-elbow cast may also be used. If the fracture is unstable, fixation with percutaneous K-wires, or even a buttress plate fixation may be necessary.

(A4)
- Median nerve compression and carpal tunnel syndrome. This is treated with carpal tunnel decompression if it does not settle rapidly.
- Sudeck's atrophy is treated by early recognition and rehabilitation with physiotherapy. The condition is prevented by early mobilisation of the fingers, elbows, shoulder and hand.
- The third complication is shortening of the radius with prominence of the ulnar styloid and a radial deviation deformity. Treatment of this condition is in most cases conservative, as in many instances it does not greatly affect the final functional outcome, particularly in elderly patients. Where shortening of the radius is such as to affect function, then either a shortening osteotomy of the ulna, or an elongation of the radius to restore length can be undertaken.

Burst fracture

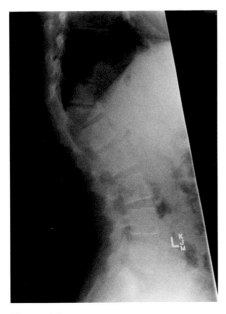

Figure 1.8

The X-ray in Figure 1.8 is that of a 30-year-old male patient who suffered an injury to his back while motocross riding. This X-ray has been taken six months after injury when the patient complained of backache. Neurologically, the patient is intact. He had been treated for six months after injury with bed rest followed by a hyper-extension cast for three months. The original X-ray at the time of the fracture showed minimal wedging of the burst fracture.

Questions

Q1 Describe the appearances of the X-ray. What type of fracture do you think the patient has suffered?

Q2 What further investigations and treatment would you recommend?

Answers

 We are seeing a wedge deformity of the 12th dorsal vertebra with a 45 degree kyphotic angulatory deformity. The appearance is of a previous unstable burst fracture with fragmentation of the anterior part of the vertebral body. The posterior column appears to have remained intact. There was probably disruption of the middle column at the time of injury. Clearly, on the basis of the description of the original X-rays after the injury, there has been a significant progression of the deformity.

- Further investigation would include CT or MRI scanning to determine the precise extent of damage, and to identify any evidence of cord deviation or compression.
- Depending on the severity of symptoms it may be necessary to consider surgical release anteriorly together with bone grafting and fusion of the spine at the affected level, D11/12. If symptoms are not severe, then a conservative approach would be indicated.

Hallux rigidus

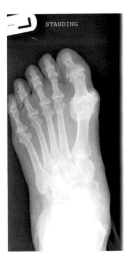

STANDING

Figure 1.9

A 50-year-old patient presents with a painful deformed foot in the region of the base of the hallux.

Questions

(Q1) Describe the X-ray appearances.

(Q2) Make a diagnosis.

(Q3) Discuss options of treatment.

Answers

A1 The X-ray appearance is of osteoarthrosis of the first metatarsophalangeal (MTP) joint or hallux rigidus, with some associated osteoarthrosis of the interphalangeal (IP) joint of the big toe.

A2 The diagnosis is therefore hallux rigidus.

A3 One treatment option is fusion of the joint. Such a fusion may be considered inappropriate in the presence of significant osteoarthrosis of the distal joint, namely the IP joint of the big toe. In this case arthroplasty with a spacer to restore functional activity to the MTP joint and relieve pain is recommended. In patients with a less active lifestyle such an option may well be considered. The third option is a Keller's excision arthroplasty. This operation involves removal of the proximal part of the proximal phalanx of the big toe, which, together with debridement and removal of osteophytes from the joint, can give rise to significant pain relief. The shortened floppy big toe is frequently unacceptable to patients if they are active, and this may therefore not be a desired option. Conservative treatment with weight loss can be used if appropriate; anti-inflammatories and analgesics and supportive footwear may be considered before a surgical solution is sought.

Fifth metacarpal fracture

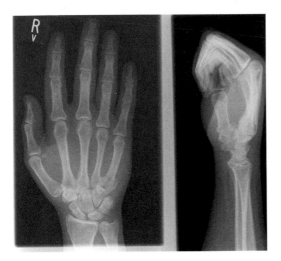

Figure 1.10

This young man struck a wall with his right fist in a fit of anger. He presented with pain in his right hand.

Questions

Q1 Describe the X-ray findings.

Q2 Discuss the management options available.

Answers

The X-ray findings show some soft tissue swelling of the hand on the ulnar side, in association with a comminuted fracture of the base of the fifth metacarpal, with involvement of the carpometacarpal joint and the joint between the fourth and fifth metacarpal bases. The overall alignment looks satisfactory, but it is not possible to say on the AP view alone whether there is a dislocation as well. The lateral view indicates that there has not been a dislocation of the proximal end of the fifth carpometacarpal joint.

- Conservative treatment with the support of a protective hand cast will allow union of the fracture to occur. Rehabilitation of hand function after a period of three weeks is to be recommended, and one would normally expect good function to be restored. Occasionally patients will go on to spontaneously fuse the fifth carpometacarpal joint after this injury, with some resultant discomfort during hand use.
- K-wire fixation of the fragments would be recommended if there is evident instability.

Hip: intertrochanteric fracture – dynamic hip screw (DHS)

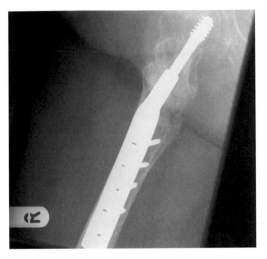

Figure 1.11

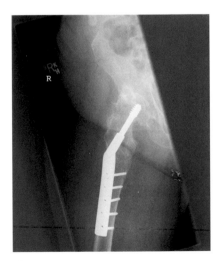

Figure 1.12

Questions

Q1 Describe the device seen on these X-rays.

Q2 Describe a classification of femoral neck fractures and discuss the importance of the classification you use.

Q3 Which particular hip fracture (Figure 1.12) do you think this device is ideally suited to?

Answers

 A dynamic hip screw.

 Hip fractures are classified as intracapsular or extracapsular fractures. The IC fractures are either subcapital or transcervical, while the EC fractures are intertrochanteric, per-trochanteric or sub-trochanteric fractures. In IC fractures there is likely to be an interference with the vascular supply to the femoral head, while with EC fractures the blood supply to the femoral head is unaffected. This distinction between EC and IC fractures will have a bearing on whether fixation or replacement is used to treat the fracture. The type of fracture, degree of displacement and patient age will all be taken into account when deciding the preferred method of treatment of the fracture.

 Intertrochanteric or per-trochanteric fracture.

Hip: sub-trochanteric fracture – intramedullary hip screw (IMHS)

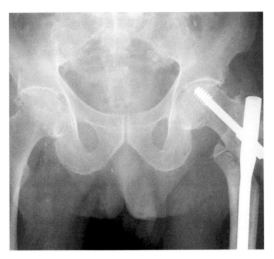

Figure 1.13

Question

Q1 Describe the device seen on these X-rays and explain why it is more suited to the fracture seen.

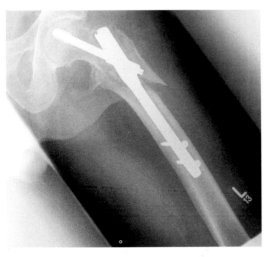

Figure 1.14

Answer

 This is an intramedullary hip screw. It consists of a screw that goes into the femoral head and an intramedullary nail stem instead of the plate in the more traditional DHS. For the more unstable sub-trochanteric fractures this device is a better option.

Osteoarthritis of the knee

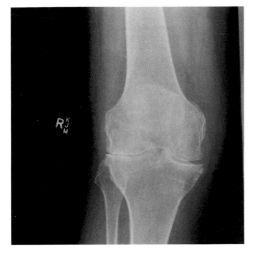

These are X-rays from an obese 55-year-old lady with a painful right knee. Examination confirms some restriction of movement, some varus deformity, and crepitus.

Questions

Q1 Describe the appearances of the X-ray.

Q2 Discuss the patient's options for treatment of this condition.

Figure 1.15

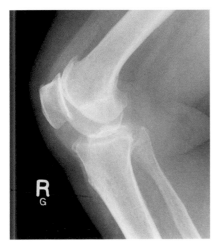

Figure 1.16

Answers

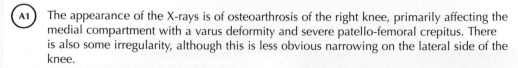

The appearance of the X-rays is of osteoarthrosis of the right knee, primarily affecting the medial compartment with a varus deformity and severe patello-femoral crepitus. There is also some irregularity, although this is less obvious narrowing on the lateral side of the knee.

Options for treatment include weight loss and conservative treatment with analgesics, anti-inflammatories and the use of a supportive cane or stick. Surgical options include arthroscopic washout of the knee, unicompartmental arthroplasty of the knee, or total knee replacement. High tibial osteotomy or double osteotomy of the knee can also be undertaken to relieve pain.

Loose Charnley total hip replacement

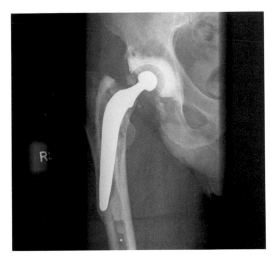

Figure 1.17

This patient underwent a Charnley total hip replacement 10 years earlier, and in the year prior to presentation complained of increasing pain in the region of the right hip replacement. Pain was mainly in the thigh on weight-bearing, and the patient had taken to using a pair of crutches to support her weight.

Questions

Q1 Describe the appearances of the X-ray.

Q2 Describe the natural progression of what is seen on the X-ray.

Q3 Discuss options of management.

Answers

(A1)   The X-ray shows a Charnley THR with a cemented acetabular and femoral component and a marker to show a cement restrictor has been used in the shaft of the femur. The Charnley femoral stem has become loose and is going into varus, with the distal tip of the prosthesis beginning to erode and protrude its way out through the femoral shaft laterally.

(A2)   The natural progression of this is to deform the lateral cortex of the femur further and ultimately probably fracture through the lateral cortex of the femur.

(A3)   Treatment options include a conservative approach with use of a stick to partially weight-bear and support the hip replacement. This option would be used if the patient was unfit for further major surgery. The other option is surgical revision of the prosthesis with a longer stem to extend below the level of the eroded bone.

Osteoarthritis of the hip

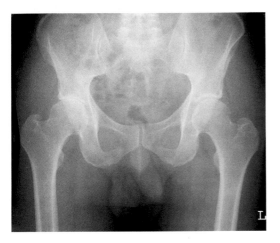

Figure 1.18

A 60-year-old male patient presented with pain in the region of the right hip, a limp, and pain at night, with pain radiating into the right groin and right buttock. A full range of movement was identified, but all extremes of movement were painful. The patient is otherwise healthy and well.

Questions

Q1   Describe the X-ray appearances.

Q2   What is the management of this problem?

Q3   List the complications of total hip replacement.

Answers

A1 This is an X-ray of a pelvis and both hips. On the left side there is a well-preserved hip joint space, no deformity and no evidence of a fracture. On the right side there is narrowing of the joint space superiorly, sclerosis of the acetabular margin, and osteophytes. These are features of primary osteoarthritis of the hip.

A2 • *Conservative treatment:* weight loss, anti-inflammatories and analgesics; use of a walking stick to support the hip; physiotherapy to mobilise the hip.
   • *Surgical treatment:* a primary total hip replacement. Another option is a resurfacing hip replacement.

A3 Instability, dislocation, early or late infection, loosening and failure/fracture of the prosthesis.

Distal radius fracture

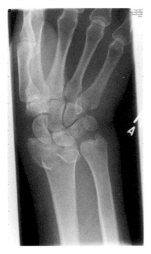

Figure 1.19

A middle-aged lady falls on to her right wrist, suffering this injury.

Questions

Q1 Describe the X-ray appearance.

Q2 What is the treatment of this injury?

Q3 List the complications of this injury and describe one of them in detail.

Answers

 There is a comminuted intra-articular fracture of the distal radius with shortening of the radius, radial deviation, and some displacement of the fragments. There is probably at least partial disruption of the distal radio-ulnar joint.

 Because of the articular and comminuted nature of this fracture, reduction and plaster immobilisation is unlikely to maintain a satisfactory position, or fixation. Percutaneous K-wires or an open reduction and plate stabilisation should be considered. At the time of surgery an accurate reduction of the wrist articular surface should be sought, and if percutaneous treatment does not achieve this, then open reduction should be considered.

- The complications are obviously median nerve compression and carpal tunnel syndrome: the patient experiences tingling or numbness in the median nerve distribution affecting the thumb, index, long and radial aspect of ring finger following injury. If this persists the treatment is carpal tunnel decompression at the time of fixation of fracture.
- Another complication is Sudeck's atrophy: the patient complains of increasing pain, stiffness and swelling in the region of the wrist, during and after plaster immobilisation. The pain is in excess of what one would expect, the skin becomes shiny, and circulatory changes appear. Once established bone scanning will confirm the diagnosis, and treatment is aggressive rehabilitation.
- The third complication is osteoarthrosis or stiffness of the wrist: because of the severe nature of the intra-articular injury in this case, stiffness of the wrist is almost inevitable. This may be in both flexion and extension as well as forearm rotation at the distal radio-ulnar joint, and osteoarthrosis of both elements of the wrist may occur later. Treatment for established osteoarthrosis of the wrist following this injury will be a fusion of the wrist if pain and a loss of strength are particular problems.

Olecranon spur

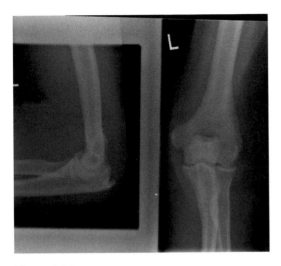

Figure 1.20

This patient presented with a large olecranon bursa and an X-ray was taken showing the appearances in Figure 1.20.

Questions

Q1 What is the treatment of an olecranon bursa?

Q2 What are the appearances on the X-ray?

Answers

 Initially treatment is conservative, by aspiration, with or without steroid injection to reduce inflammation. Ultimately if there is recurrence, consider excision.

 There is a large olecranon spur visible on X-ray. This may or may not be related to the occurrence of a bursitis or olecranon bursa. If surgery for a bursa is to be considered, the olecranon spur should be excised at the same time. If the spur is asymptomatic and the bursitis resolves without recurrence, then the spur does not need excision.

Hip osteotomy for congenital hip dysplasia/DDH

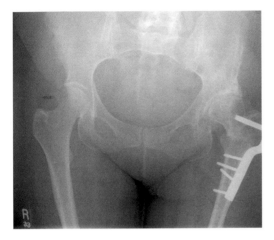

Figure 1.21

Questions

Q1 Describe the appearance of this X-ray.

Q2 What is the device that is seen in the left hip?

Q3 What operation has been undertaken?

Answers

A1 The description is an X-ray of the pelvis with a normal right hip. On the left side there is osteoarthrosis of a deformed left hip, with flattening of the acetabulum and femoral head, and lateral displacement of the head consistent with congenital hip dysplasia.

A2 On the left side there is a device which one can describe as an osteotomy plate and screws.

A3 A femoral neck osteotomy has been performed.

Clavicle fracture (1)

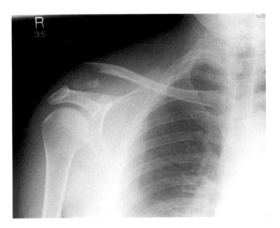

Figure 1.22

This patient fell off his bicycle suffering an injury to his right shoulder. Examination showed tenderness and deformity in the region of the outer end of the clavicle, and X-rays are as shown.

Questions

Q1 Describe the injury as seen.

Q2 Describe a classification of fractures of the outer end of the clavicle.

Q3 Describe two of the complications of this fracture.

Answers

A1 There is a displaced fracture of the outer end of the clavicle, which does not involve the acromioclavicular joint. There is superior displacement of the proximal fragment. The remainder of the shaft of the clavicle looks normal. It is likely that there has been at least a partial disruption of the vertical coraco-clavicular ligament.

A2 *The Neer classification:*
- Grade I is an undisplaced non-articular fracture of the outer end of the clavicle, without disruption of the coraco-clavicular ligaments
- Grade II is a non-articular displaced fracture of the outer end of the clavicle
- Grade III is an intra-articular fracture of the outer end of the clavicle.

A3
- Non-union: there is a high incidence of non-union of this fracture, which may, or may not be symptomatic. If it is symptomatic, then a reduction of the fracture, together with bone grafting and plating may be necessary to achieve union.
- The second complication is tenting or perforation of the skin, with a potential for the fracture to become compound because of the sharp nature of the proximal fragment and its upward displacement. In association with this complication is a perforation of the deltoid or delto-trapezius, which contributes to the non-union. The treatment for this is a reduction of the fracture, release of the overlying skin, and repair of the deltoid or delto-trapezius injury.

Hallux valgus

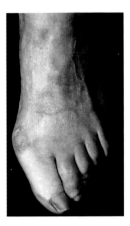

Figure 1.23

Questions

Q1 Describe the clinical findings.

Q2 What are the predisposing factors and aetiology of this condition?

Q3 What is a bunionette?

Q4 What treatment options are available for this problem?

Answers

 • There is marked hallux valgus.
 • Prominence of the first metatarsal head.
 • Widening of the forefoot.
 • Bunion.
 • Crowding and deformity – overlapping of the second toe and hammer toes.

 Predisposing factors are essentially unknown but:
 • there is a strong familial trait
 • there is increased incidence in people who wear enclosed footwear – it is rarely seen in those who have never worn shoes
 • it is associated with rheumatoid arthritis
 • it is secondary to metatarsus primus varus which itself may be congenital or secondary to loss of muscle tone with age.

 A bunionette is a prominence of the medial aspect of the first metatarsal head.

 • *Non-surgical*:
   – appropriate footwear – wide shoe, wide toe box and protective padding over prominences
   – surgeon to follow-up to examine footwear and wear patterns
   – physiotherapy.
 • *Surgical*: several options are available; it depends on the wishes of the patient, level of activity and state of peripheral vascular system. Options include:
   – bunionectomy
   – first metatarsal realignment osteotomy
   – excision arthroplasty (Keller's procedure)
   – fusion – for degenerative joint disease.

Posterior dislocation of the shoulder (1)

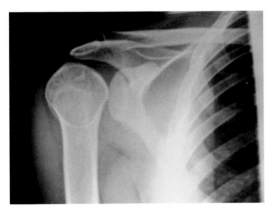

Figure 1.24

Questions

Q1 What sign does this X-ray show and what is the diagnosis?

Q2 What is the mechanism of injury and what co-morbidity normally predisposes to this problem?

Q3 Why can this view on the X-ray be misleading?

Q4 How would you correct the problem?

Q5 What are the commonest complications of this condition?

Q6 What are the other forms of this type of injury to the joint affected? Which is the commonest one seen?

Answers

(A1) The Light Bulb Sign. The diagnosis is posterior dislocation of the right shoulder.

(A2) In posterior dislocation the humeral head lies posterior to the glenoid. It usually results from a fall onto an outstretched internally rotated hand or direct blow to the front of the shoulder following an electric shock or fit causing involuntary muscle contractions. Epilepsy predisposes to the problem.

(A3) Often the AP view looks normal. Lateral views are required to show the dislocation.

(A4)
- Reduction of dislocation: apply traction to the arm with the elbow flexed and arm abducted to 90 degrees. Slowly externally rotate. The arm is then immobilised in a sling for one month. Older patients are mobilised within two weeks to prevent stiffness and loss of function. The patient will be left with a permanently restricted range of movement – due to adhesions forming between the capsule and humeral head. The mainstay of treatment is graduated shoulder physiotherapy.
- Steroid injections.
- Manipulation under anaesthetic.
- There is a 50% chance of recurrence within two years.
- If further dislocations occur (>4 times) reconstructive surgery should be considered.

(A5) Divide into early and late.
- *Early*:
  - axillary nerve palsy, suprascapular nerve or posterior cord of brachial plexus injury
  - arterial injury – axillary artery
  - supraspinatus tear
  - fracture of the surgical neck or greater tuberosity of the humerus.
- *Late*:
  - joint stiffness
  - recurrent dislocation.

(A6) Anterior dislocation and luxatio erecta. Anterior dislocation is by far the commonest.

Balanced traction of the fractured femur

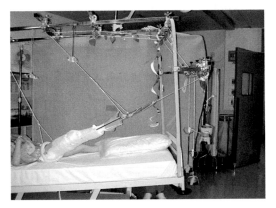

Figure 1.25

Questions

Q1 Describe the isolated injury that is being treated.

Q2 List the complications that can occur with this method of treatment.

Q3 Describe the treatment for a similar fracture in a child of one year and in an adult.

The picture shows a 7-year-old child in balanced traction.

Answers

 The picture shows a child in balanced traction for a fracture of the shaft of femur.

 The complications that need to be considered with this treatment for this injury are:
- excessive traction resulting in lengthening of the femur during fracture healing
- poor control of the position of the fracture with dropping posteriorly of the proximal end of the distal fragment of the femur
- skin exfoliation and ulceration from the skin traction
- neurovascular complications, in particular a foot drop either as a result of pressure over the neck of the fibula or excessive traction
- a pressure sore in the region of the ring of the Thomas' splint either in the groin or in the gluteal fold, due to the use of a splint in which the ring is too tight
- a pressure sore at the top of the sling used to support the back of the thigh proximally.

- A similar fracture of the shaft of the femur in a one-year old child can be treated with a plaster cast hip spica, or with Gallows traction.
- A similar fracture in an adult can be treated with balanced traction or nowadays is more likely to be treated with internal fixation using a locked nail or a plate.

Clavicle fracture (2)

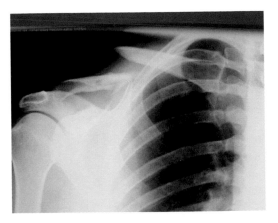

Figure 1.26

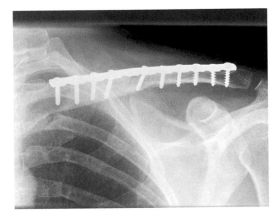

Figure 1.27

The patient sustained a displaced midshaft fracture of the right clavicle in a rugby tackle. X-rays are shown.

Questions

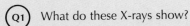 **Q1** What do these X-rays show?

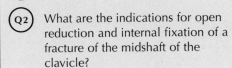 **Q2** What are the indications for open reduction and internal fixation of a fracture of the midshaft of the clavicle?

Answers

  • Displaced midshaft clavicle fracture (Figure 1.26).
  • Plate fixation of midshaft clavicle fracture (Figure 1.27).

  • Neurovascular damage: after exploration of the neurovascular injury, fixation of the clavicle gives a more stable skeleton to protect the repair.
  • A compound fracture of the clavicle may require fixation after thorough debridement of the wound.
  • A closed fracture is at risk of becoming an open fracture by reason of a displaced fragment that tents the skin.
  • Severe displacement of a midshaft fracture with obvious significant soft tissue interposition.
  • A symptomatic non-union of a fracture of the clavicle is an indication for open reduction, excision of the non-union, plating and grafting of the clavicle.

Segmental fracture of the radial head

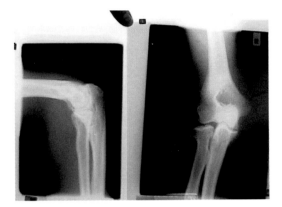

Figure 1.28

A 50-year-old female patient suffers an injury to her right elbow in a fall. Her X-ray is shown.

Questions

Q1 Describe the injury as seen on the X-ray.

Q2 The patient has swelling and pain as well as a markedly restricted range of movement. Describe what measures you would take in the accident and emergency department to alleviate the pain.

Q3 What form of immobilisation or splintage would you recommend?

Q4 What is the most common long-term complication following this injury and how is it avoided?

Answers

(A1) A segmental fracture of the radial head with minor displacement (Mason Grade I). There is no evidence of dislocation of the elbow joint.

(A2) Analgesics, anti-inflammatories and aspiration of the haemarthrosis.

(A3) A broad arm sling may be sufficient if pain after aspiration is not severe. Application of a back splint for support and pain relief may be considered. Follow-up with physiotherapy to avoid later stiffness.

(A4) Elbow stiffness is the commonest complication. It is avoided by early pain relief as described above, early mobilisation once pain relief is achieved, and early return to normal activities as pain and movement allow.

Midshaft fracture of the humerus

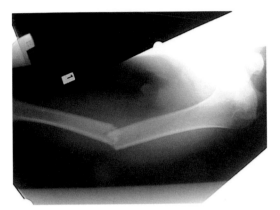

Figure 1.29

A 45-year-old female patient fell downstairs at home and suffered a midshaft fracture of the left humerus as shown in the figures.

Questions

Q1 List the most likely local early complications of this injury.

Q2 Describe the treatment alternatives for this fracture.

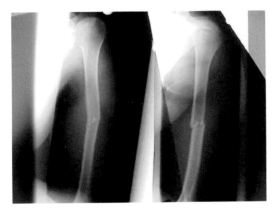

Figure 1.30

Answers

 Radial nerve palsy.

- Hanging cast.
- Intramedullary locked nail.
- Open reduction and plate fixation.

Anterior dislocation of the shoulder

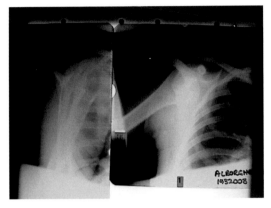

Figure 1.31

The patient is a 25-year-old female who suffered an injury to her right shoulder in a fall. X-rays are as shown.

Questions

Q1 Describe the nature of this bony injury.

Q2 In considering any question of a dislocation, specify the direction and why you consider it to be so.

Q3 Indicate what neurological injury may occur as a result of this injury.

Q4 Describe one method of treatment for this injury.

Answers

(A1) This is an anterior dislocation of the shoulder without evidence of a fracture.

(A2) It is anterior because on the lateral scapular X-ray the humeral head is seen to lie anteriorly under the coracoid process.

(A3) The likely nerve injuries that occur with this injury are an injury to the axillary nerve and an injury to C5 and C6 nerve roots of the brachial plexus.

(A4) Manipulative reduction under sedation and analgesia or under general anaesthesia, using Kocher's method of adduction, external rotation followed by internal rotation and bringing the arm back to the side by internal rotation.

Humeral surgical neck fracture

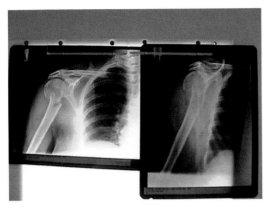

Figure 1.32

The clinical history is of an 85-year-old (right-handed?) patient who takes a fall and suffers the injury that is seen on the X-rays.

Questions

(Q1) Describe the fracture.

(Q2) Outline one method of treatment.

Answers

 The fracture is a moderately displaced humeral surgical neck fracture, with undisplaced comminution of the proximal fragment.

 Treatment options include a collar and cuff, particularly if the patient is sedentary or unfit; or intramedullary nailing or other method of fixation if the patient is very active and requires the aggressive use of this, the dominant arm.

Clavicle fracture (3)

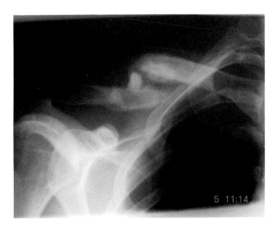

Figure 1.33

This X-ray of the right clavicle was taken six months after the patient, a 35-year-old male, had fallen from a motorcycle and suffered this injury to his clavicle.

Questions

Q1 Describe the injury, and the X-ray appearance considering the interval since injury.

Q2 The patient complains of considerable discomfort and pain around the region of the fracture, is unhappy with the deformity it gives, and complains of weakness of shoulder movement. Describe the various options for treatment in this case.

Answers

A1   The X-ray shows a displaced midshaft fracture of the right clavicle with a hypertrophic non-union.

A2   In the context of the symptoms of which he is complaining, the correct treatment would be open reduction, excision of the non-union, fixation of the fracture with a rigid plate and application of bone graft.

Elbow dislocation

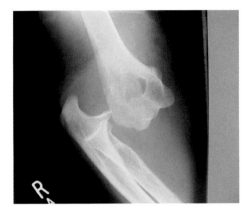

Figure 1.34

Figures 1.34 and 1.35 show complete postero-medial dislocation of an elbow. The patient is a 31-year-old male who fell off a ladder sustaining an injury to his right elbow. Gross deformity of the right elbow was noted, severe swelling was present, circulation was poor, with a cold hand, and there was paraesthesia over the distribution of the ulnar nerve.

Questions

Q1 Describe the injury.

Q2 Describe the urgent management of this problem.

Q3 In the event that, following reduction, the circulation is not restored, describe the next stage of management.

Q4 List the long-term complications of this injury.

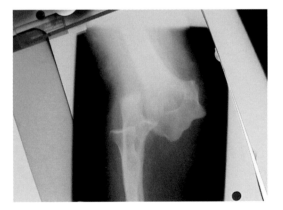

Figure 1.35

Answers

 Severe complete postero-medial dislocation of the elbow without an associated fracture.

 • Analgesia.
• Assessment of neurovascular status.
• Urgent surgery to reduce the dislocation.
• Post-reduction X-ray and check of neurovascular status.

 Doppler ultrasound may be used to detect circulatory function, followed by intra-operative angiogram and appropriate exploration and repair of the vessel if necessary.

 • Recurrent instability.
• Elbow stiffness.
• Restricted range of movement.
• Persistence of neurological dysfunction.

Arthrogram of the shoulder

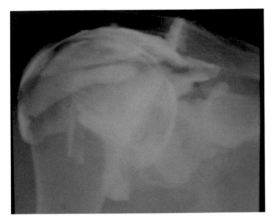

Figure 1.36

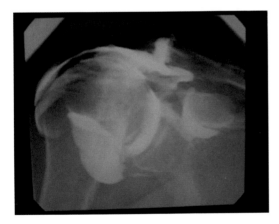

Figure 1.37

Questions

Q1 What are these radiographs?

Q2 What do they show?

Answers

 Arthrogram of the right shoulder.

 A full-thickness rotator cuff tear with contrast exuding into the acromioclavicular joint (the Geiser sign). The significance of the Geiser sign is a complete disruption of the inferior acromioclavicular ligament, usually indicating a large full-thickness rotator cuff tear.

Proximal humeral fracture

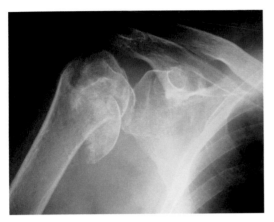

Figure 1.38

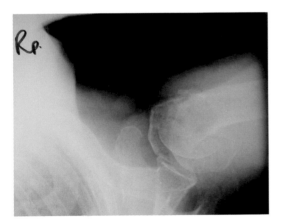

Figure 1.39

Questions

Q1 What is the nature of the injury seen on these X-rays?

Q2 What further investigation would be worthwhile before making a final decision on treatment?

Q3 List the management options for this injury with an indication as to why each option should be considered.

Answers

 A1 This is a comminuted head-splitting fracture of the proximal right humerus, with subluxation or dislocation of at least part of the humeral head.

 A2 CT scan.

 A3
- Open reduction and internal fixation. This could be considered if the CT scan demonstrates a sufficiently large fragment of the humeral head as a single segment.
- Hemi-arthroplasty. This is most likely to be the optimum method of treatment, as the CT scan is likely to show a comminuted head-splitting fracture of the proximal humerus.

Knee trauma

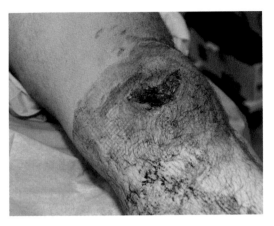

Figure 1.40

The patient is a 43-year-old driver of a car involved in a head-on collision. The only visible injury is that seen in the Figure.

Questions

Q1 In assessing this injury, indicate what structures are likely to have been damaged and need careful assessment.

Q2 What other joint in the limb may have sustained a significant injury, and what specific injury will that be?

Answers

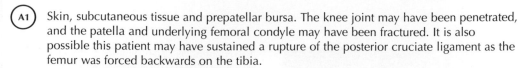

A1 Skin, subcutaneous tissue and prepatellar bursa. The knee joint may have been penetrated, and the patella and underlying femoral condyle may have been fractured. It is also possible this patient may have sustained a rupture of the posterior cruciate ligament as the femur was forced backwards on the tibia.

A2 The hip proximal to the knee, and the injury would be a posterior dislocation or fracture dislocation of the hip.

Supracondylar fracture

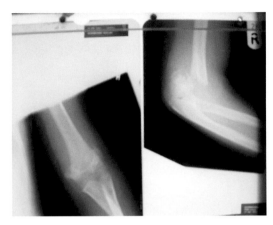

Figure 1.41

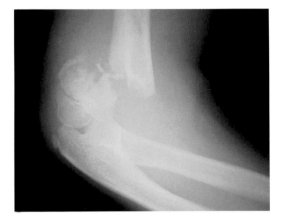

Figure 1.42

Questions

Q1 Describe the injury as seen on X-ray.

Q2 Aside from local swelling, what other physical findings should be urgently assessed?

Q3 In the event that a vascular occlusion results in significant compromise to the vascular supply of the limb following this injury, a Volkman's ischaemic contracture may occur. Describe the clinical features of a Volkman's ischaemic contracture:
(a) in its early developing stage
(b) in its late stage.

Q4 Describe the treatment of this injury.

Answers

(A1) Displaced posterior extension-type supracondylar fracture of the right elbow in a child.

(A2) The radial pulse.

(A3) (a) The physical finding suggesting the development of a Volkman's ischaemic contracture is pain experienced in the forearm during passive extension of the fingers.

(b) An established Volkman's ischaemic contracture results in shortening of the length of soft tissue relative to the bones and joints. This results in flexion of the fingers when the wrist is straight or extended, and the fingers can only be extended in the presence of a flexed wrist.

(A4) Urgent reduction of the fracture and re-establishment of circulatory function.

Lateral condylar fracture of the humerus

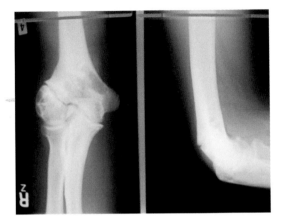

Figure 1.43

This patient suffered a fracture of the lateral condyle of the right humerus in a fall from a bicycle ten years earlier. His presenting symptoms were of a significantly reduced range of movement in his elbow, in association with wasting of the small muscles of the hand (excluding the thenar muscles), and paraesthesia affecting the little and middle finger and ulnar side of the ring finger.

Questions

Q1 What is the diagnosis?

Q2 What is the treatment for this condition?

Answers

- Un-united fracture of the lateral condyle, joint irregularity and arthrosis of the elbow.
- A tardy ulnar nerve palsy.

- Nerve conduction studies may be considered to establish the severity of the nerve problem.
- Ulnar nerve release with possible epicondylectomy or anterior transposition.
- Consideration needs to be given to whether a re-establishment of an appropriate joint surface alignment may improve movement.
- An attempt may be made to consider achieving union of the fracture by excision and bone grafting.
- If elbow joint arthritis is sufficiently severe, an elbow replacement may be considered.

Posterior dislocation of the shoulder (2)

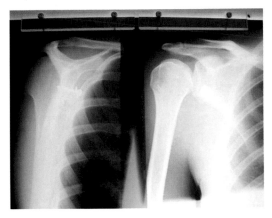

Figure 1.44

Questions

Q1   What is the clinical diagnosis of these X-rays?

Q2   Is there any evidence to suggest that this patient has had previous surgery, and if so, what do you think the surgery was?

Q3   What is the treatment for this condition?

Answers

(A1) A posterior dislocation of the right shoulder.

(A2) The presence of a screw and washer in the glenoid going from anterior to posterior suggests a previous anterior stabilisation of the shoulder.

(A3) Manipulative reduction of the dislocation, check of X-ray, splintage in external rotation, and consideration of further stabilisation if recurrent dislocation occurs.

Luxatio erecta of the shoulder

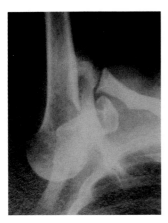

Figure 1.45

The patient slipped off a ladder and grabbed a ladder rung on his way down. He experienced sudden severe pain in his right shoulder and arm, and found his arm locked above his head. On arrival at the casualty department his arm was still held in abduction and elevation, and the X-ray is shown.

Questions

Q1 Describe the X-ray findings, and make your diagnosis on that basis.

Q2 Describe the treatment for this injury.

Q3 What important local complications are associated with this injury?

Answers

A1 True inferior dislocation with abduction of the arm (luxatio erecta) with incidental acromioclavicular joint arthrosis.

A2 Immediate reduction under anaesthetic with relaxation by gentle traction and manipulation with an image intensifier to confirm reduction.

A3
- Rotator cuff tear.
- Axillary nerve palsy.
- Fracture of the proximal humerus during attempted reduction.
- Arterial and brachial plexus injury.

Fracture dislocation of the shoulder (2)

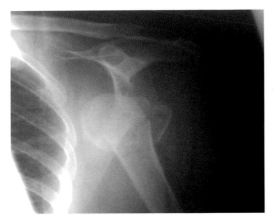

Figure 1.46

Questions

Q1 Describe the radiological features on this X-ray.

Q2 Describe the treatment for this injury.

Q3 What is the most serious risk of manipulative reduction of this fracture dislocation?

Answers

(A1)   Dislocation of the glenohumeral joint with a fracture of the greater tuberosity and fracture of the surgical neck of the humerus (three-part fracture dislocation).

(A2)   Manipulative reduction under a full general anaesthetic and relaxation with the image intensifier.

(A3)   Extension of the fracture lines leaving the humeral head in a dislocated position while the humeral shaft returns into its normal alignment.

Osteoathritis of the shoulder (1)

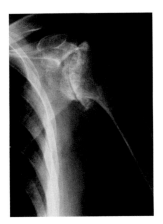

Figure 1.47

This 60-year-old patient complained of increasing pain and stiffness in his left shoulder. Examination confirmed equal restriction of both passive and active movement to less than 50% of normal. An X-ray of his left shoulder is seen.

Questions

Q1 Describe the findings on the X-ray.

Q2 What is the treatment of choice for this condition in an otherwise active, healthy man who has no evidence of systemic or local infection?

Answers

 Loss of joint space, osteophytes, subchondral cysts and subchondral sclerosis indicating typical osteoarthrosis of the glenohumeral joint.

 Shoulder replacement.

Osteoarthritis of the shoulder (2)

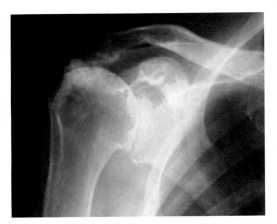

Figure 1.48

This is the X-ray of a 70-year-old female with a painful shoulder. She has virtually no active movement, but passive movement is full.

Questions

Q1 Indicate the significance of the greater passive over active movement.

Q2 Describe the X-ray features.

Q3 What is the diagnosis based on this X-ray?

Q4 What further investigations are necessary to confirm the diagnosis?

Q5 Justify your response to the previous question.

Answers

(A1) The presence of a greater passive range of movement over active range of movement indicates a neuromuscular/tendonous problem.

(A2) Narrowing of the subacromial space, the four features of osteoarthrosis, and upward subluxation of the humeral head.

(A3) Osteoarthrosis secondary to a complete rotator cuff absence.

(A4) None.

(A5) All investigations will confirm a significant full-thickness global cuff tear, which examination of the X-ray already diagnosed. There is therefore no justification for undertaking any further investigations in the context of what treatment should be undertaken.

Locked posterior dislocation

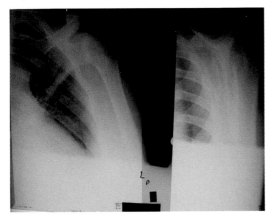

Figure 1.49

The patient is a 25-year-old male with diabetes, who complained of sudden onset of severe pain in his left shoulder at 2 am. The pain woke him from his sleep. Examination was not possible as he was in too much pain on attendance at the accident and emergency department, and X-rays showed these findings.

Questions

Q1 Describe the X-ray findings and make a diagnosis.

Q2 What are the clinical features of a locked posterior dislocation?

Q3 What further investigations would you ask for, and what is the treatment for this condition?

Answers

(A1) A locked posterior dislocation of the left shoulder.

(A2) Prominence posteriorly of the humeral head, hollowing anteriorly, and fixed internal rotation with inability to elevate the hand away from the trunk.

(A3) • A CT scan will demonstrate the presence of a locked posterior dislocation, the presence or absence of any fracture lines, and the severity and extent of the locking. This investigation will give a good indication as to whether a closed reduction may be possible.
• Treatment of the condition is to achieve a reduction by a closed or open operative means, and depending on the size of the defect, consider stabilisation or hemi-arthroplasty.

Off-ended fracture in a child

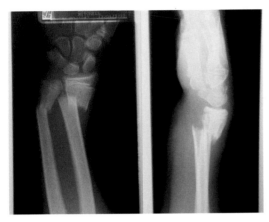

Figure 1.50

The child presented to the accident and emergency department having fallen from his bicycle, with a painful deformed and swollen wrist. X-rays are shown.

Questions

(Q1) Describe the X-rays.

(Q2) Discuss the management of this problem.

Answers

 The X-rays show off-ended fractures of the radius and ulna within approximately 4 cm of the distal end, with some radial and dorsal deviation (a childhood Colles' fracture would be an acceptable description).

 Management of this injury is by manipulation and reduction of the fracture. It may occasionally be necessary to use K-wire fixation if the fracture is unstable after reduction.

Radio-carpal dislocation

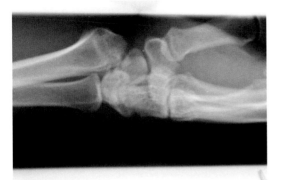

Figure 1.51

A 40-year-old male patient fell 10 ft off a roof, landing onto his outstretched hand. Clinically a significant and severe deformity and swelling was noted on admission, and the X-rays are as shown.

Questions

Q1 Describe the injury that this man has sustained.

Q2 Describe the treatment that should be considered.

Q3 What early and late complications are likely to occur?

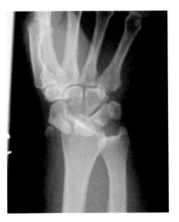

Figure 1.52

Answers

(A1)   The injury is a radio-carpal dislocation with a fracture of the radial and ulnar styloids.

(A2)   The treatment is urgent reduction with stabilisation either by fixation of the styloid processes or by transradio-carpal K-wiring.

(A3)   Early complications include carpal tunnel median nerve compression and radial artery injury, and late complications include radio-carpal instability and wrist stiffness.

Bone tumours

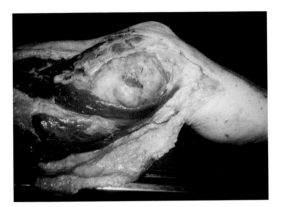

Figure 1.53

Questions

Q1 What is demonstrated in Figure 1.53? Define a bone tumour.

Q2 What are the causes of bone tumours?

Q3 Discuss the incidence of bone tumours.

Q4 What are the symptoms of a bone tumour?

Q5 What are the diagnostic tests available to evaluate bone tumours? What is the staging work-up for bone tumours? Discuss the importance of taking biopsies of the lesions.

Q6 What are the subtypes of surgical resections?

Q7 What are the treatment options available?

Q8 What is the prognosis?

Q9 What are the complications of a bone tumour?

Q10 What are the general principles of fixation of pathological fractures?

Q11 Discuss limb salvage surgery and its principles.

Answers

 A large bone tumour involving the lower end of the femur. A bone tumour is an abnormal growth of cells within the bone that may be benign or malignant.

- Idiopathic: in most cases no specific cause is found.
- They often arise in areas of rapid growth.
- Inherited mutations.
- Increased in families with familial cancer syndromes.
- Trauma.
- Radiation/industrial exposure to radium.

 Bone tumours may be benign or malignant.

Benign tumours
Benign bone tumours include non-ossifying fibroma, unicameral (simple) bone cyst, osteochondroma, giant cell tumour, enchondroma and fibrous dysplasia.
Osteochondromas are the most common benign bone tumours and occur most often in people between the ages of 10 and 20 years. Some benign bone tumours do not require treatment and may disappear with time. These benign tumours are monitored periodically by X-ray.

Malignant tumours
Malignant bone tumours occur as a primary bone tumour or as metastases.

Primary tumours
Primary bone tumours are rare (less than 1% of all malignant tumours) and are most common in young men. The four most common types of primary bone cancer are:
- *multiple myeloma*, the most common primary bone cancer. This is a malignant tumour of bone marrow. It affects approximately 20 people per million each year. Most cases are seen in patients aged 50 to 70 years. Any bone can be involved
- *osteosarcoma* is the second most common bone cancer. It occurs in two or three new people per million people each year. Most cases occur in teenagers. Most tumours occur around the knee. Other common locations include the hip and shoulder
- *Ewing's sarcoma* most commonly occurs between ages 5 and 20 years. The most common locations are the upper and lower leg, pelvis, upper arm and ribs
- *chondrosarcoma* occurs most commonly in patients aged 40 to 70 years. Most cases occur around the hip and pelvis or shoulder.

Secondary tumours
The most common cancers that spread to the bone are of the breast, lung, prostate, kidney, and thyroid. These forms of cancer usually affect older people. The incidence of bone cancer in children is approximately five cases per million children each year.

- Bone pain, may be worse at night. The pain is generally described as a dull ache.
- Occasionally a mass and swelling can be felt at the tumour site.
- Bone fracture, especially fracture from trivial trauma.
- Rarely it can also cause fevers and night sweats.
- Some benign tumours have no symptoms.

- X-ray.
- MRI.
- Bone scan showing the size and location of the tumour.
- Altered biochemical bone profiles: PTH, calcium (serum and ionised) and alkaline phosphatase.
- Trucut or open biopsy.

The basic staging work-up should include high-quality plain radiographs of the affected bone or soft tissue area, an MRI study of the entire tumour and nearby anatomical structures, a CT scan of the chest, a whole-body technetium bone scan, and a biopsy of the tumour. Evaluation of the images by an experienced orthopaedic oncologist or musculoskeletal radiologist can often narrow the differential diagnosis down to one or two entities. Sometimes the tumour may be found to be benign, and multiple expensive tests may never be needed.

Biopsy is not a part of the initial management of these lesions and is usually the last step in the work-up. Except in rare instances, the surgeon who will be doing the definitive surgery should perform the biopsy. Biopsy-related complications have been shown to lead to an amputation being required in cases where the limb might otherwise have been salvaged. The best location and method for the biopsy is selected based on the results of the staging work-up. The biopsy site must be carefully planned and located along so-called 'limb salvage lines', so that the entire biopsy track can be excised en bloc with the tumour if limb salvage surgery becomes necessary.

Resections can be classified based on the type of margin achieved during surgery as follows:
- *an intralesional resection* is created if the tumour is entered or cut into at any point during surgery
- *a marginal resection* is created when the surgical dissection extends into or through the abnormal, reactive tissues that surround the tumour but are not actually a part of the tumour, the so-called 'reactive zone'
- *a wide local excision/resection* is created when the reactive zone is not entered, but instead the dissection is through entirely normal tissues, and a cuff of normal tissue is left on all sides of the tumour
- *a radical resection* is resection of the entire bony or myofascial compartment or compartments containing the tumour.

Exactly what constitutes an adequate margin in any particular case remains controversial. For high-grade sarcomas, a wide margin is considered adequate and will achieve successful control of the primary tumour approximately 95% of the time, whereas marginal or intralesional margins are associated with frequent local recurrence and poor outcomes. In low-grade tumours or in high-grade tumours where pre-operative radiation therapy has been given, a minimal margin may be adequate.

Benign tumours
- May not require treatment but may be assessed periodically to check for progression or regression.
- Surgical removal.

Malignant tumours
- Primary malignant tumours are rare and require treatment at centres with experience of treating these cancers.
- Tumours that have spread to bone depend upon the primary tissue or organ involved.

- Radiation therapy with chemotherapy or hormone therapy is commonly used.
- A combination of chemotherapy and surgery is usually necessary.
- Limb salvage surgery involves the removal of the tumorous section of the bone with a clear margin preserving nearby muscles, tendons, nerves and blood vessels. The excised bone is replaced with a metallic implant (prosthesis) or bone transplant.
- Amputation removes all or part of a limb when the tumour is large and/or nerves and blood vessels are involved.
- Radiation therapy may be needed before or after surgery.

 The prognosis varies depending on the type of tumour. The outcome is expected to be good for people with benign tumours, although some types of benign tumour may eventually become malignant.

With malignant bone tumours that have not spread, most patients achieve a cure. The cure rate depends on the type of cancer, location, size, and other factors.

A9
- Pain.
- Pathological fracture.
- Function may be reduced depending on the extent of the tumour.
- Spread of the cancer to other nearby/distant tissues (metastasis).
- Side-effects of chemotherapy.

A10 Pathological fractures create a serious morbidity in patients with metastatic bone disease. Orthopaedic surgeons who treat patients with metastatic skeletal lesions should focus on proactive treatments designed to prevent pathological fractures before they occur. Prevention of pathological fractures results in better patient outcome, lower cost, and less-difficult operative procedures. For this reason, it is critical to identify both patients and skeletal lesions that are at increased risk of pathological fracture.
- The risk of pathological fracture increases with the duration of metastatic disease. Hence a patient who has a relatively long survival is more likely to sustain a pathological fracture.
- Purely lytic metastases are more likely to fracture than those that are blastic or mixed lytic and blastic.
- Blastic metastases are less susceptible to fracture, but blastic lesions have been shown to decrease the longitudinal stiffness of bone blastic lesions in high-risk areas such as the proximal femur, and have a high rate of fracture.
- Irradiation of metastatic bone lesions also appears to increase the risk of pathological fracture as it causes temporary softening of the bone at the tumour site and failure of re-ossification after treatment. Patients who have low bone density due to hormone modification therapies should be considered at increased risk for fracture.
- Unusually expansile and destructive lesions are an increased risk for pathological fracture.
- Pain may be a valuable sign of decreased mechanical strength of bone and increased fracture risk.
- Patients with greater than 50% of bony cortical involvement usually develop a fracture.
- Location of lesion: any involvement of cortex in the sub-trochanteric region of femur increases fracture risk.

• Every patient with a malignant tumour of the extremity should be considered for limb salvage if the tumour can be removed with an adequate margin and the resulting limb is worth saving.

- An adequate margin is one that results in an acceptably low rate of local recurrence of the tumour.

- A salvaged limb must provide a reasonable degree of function, cosmetic appearance, minimal amount of pain, and be durable enough to withstand the demands of normal daily activities.

- The patient's prognosis has a limited impact on the decision to perform limb salvage surgery as the ability to predict the survival of any particular patient is quite limited, and some of the most valuable information is unavailable until after the limb salvage procedure is completed.

- Limb salvage can be combined with metastasectomy.

- For patients with uncontrollable disease, limb salvage should be considered if the surgery could be accomplished with minimum morbidity and rapid return to function. These patients can enjoy relief from pain, improved quality of life, and intact body image, even if they may not survive long term.

- Barriers to limb salvage include poorly placed biopsy incisions, major vascular involvement, encasement of a major motor nerve or pathological fracture of the involved bone.

- The four key components needed for a viable limb are the bone, the nerves, the vessels, and the soft tissue envelope. If just one or two of these key components must be resected in order to obtain an adequate margin around the tumour, then the limb may be salvageable. If three of these key components are involved, limb salvage is probably not worth considering.

Your revision notes:

Osteomyelitis (of the clavicle)

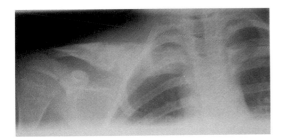

Figure 1.54

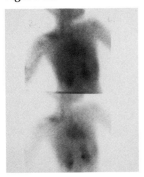

Figure 1.55

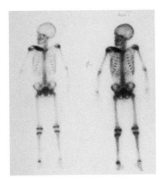

Figure 1.56

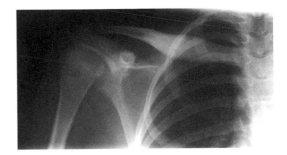

Figure 1.57

Questions

Q1 What is the most likely diagnosis (Figure 1.54) in this patient with a six-month history of a discharging sinus over his right clavicle? What is the definition of the underlying problem?

Q2 What are the classic pathological sequelae of this condition?

Q3 What are the typical clinical features?

Q4 What investigations will you instigate?

Q5 What are the differential diagnoses?

Q6 What are the common infecting organisms?

Q7 What are the late complications?

Q8 What are the principles of treatment?

Answers

  The diagnosis is osteomyelitis of the clavicle. The underlying problem is inflammation of bone or bone marrow.

- Suppuration with pus in the bone marrow.
- Sequestrum: dead bone within the periosteum forms the inner part of the infected bone and marrow.
- Involucrum: periosteal reaction to form new bone that envelopes the infected site and contains it.
- Cloacae: holes in the involucrum through which pus formed in the medulla discharges.
- Sinus: the track for drainage from cloaca to the skin.
- Septicaemia.

- Increasing severity of pain.
- Localised bony tenderness.
- Systemic toxicity and pyrexia.
- Joint effusion – adjacent joints may contain an effusion, however the joint will not be tender and some movement is possible as opposed to an infective arthritis in which no movement is permitted.

- Plain X-ray (see Figure 1.55 top).
  Note there are no radiological features in the first few days (Figure 1.57). After 10 days, periosteal elevation may be seen with new bone formation.
- Isotope bone scan (early and delayed phases) showing increased uptake in the right clavicle – where the site of infection is.
- Isotope bone scanning: this is useful in areas of difficult localisation where bone infection is to be distinguished from adjacent soft tissue infection and where joint infection must be distinguished from transient synovitis.
- Blood cultures: taken before commencing antibiotics.
- FBC, CRP, ESR to monitor progress.

- Acute suppurative arthritis: distinguish joint pain from bone pain.
- Acute rheumatic arthritis: usually polyarticular.
- Haemarthrosis, e.g. haemophilia.
- Scurvy: subperiosteal haematoma mimics pain.
- Bone infarct secondary to sickle crisis.
- Ewing's sarcoma.

- *Staphylococcus aureus.*
- *E. coli.*
- *Streptococci* spp.
- Bowel organisms such as pseudomonas.
- Salmonella especially in patients with sickle cell disease.

- Amyloidosis.
- Malignant change in the sinus – Marjolin's ulcer.
- Septicaemia and pyaemia.
- Suppurative arthritis.

Intravenous antibiotics and surgical evacuation of the abscess are required. A chronic abscess will not resolve if foreign bodies such as prostheses, mesh, or bone sequestra remain.

Paget's disease of the bone

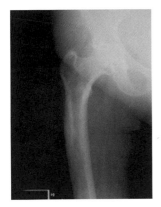

Figure 1.58

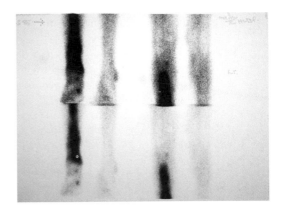

Figure 1.61

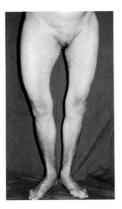

Figure 1.59

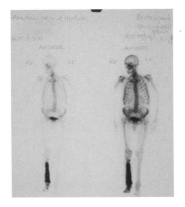

Figure 1.60

Questions

Q1 Describe what you see in the photograph (Figure 1.59) and describe the radiological changes in Figure 1.58.

Q2 What is the diagnosis?

Q3 What is the pathology of this condition?

Q4 What investigations would confirm the diagnosis?

Q5 What are the potential complications of this disease?

Q6 What stages can this disease be divided into?

Q7 How can this condition be treated?

Answers

 • Bowing of the right femur.
• The femur shows thickening, with sclerotic changes and bowing.

 Paget's disease of the bone.

 • Paget's disease is a bone disorder caused by a slow viral infection of osteoblasts and then osteoclasts by paramyxovirus.
• There is increased bone turnover with excessive osteoclastic resorption but also equivalent osteoblastic activity to replace bone. The bone formed is soft and lacks normal mineralisation.
• It usually begins in mid-adulthood and is more common in white people in Europe and Australia.

 • Very high levels of serum alkaline phosphatase due to excess bone turnover.
• A mixture of osteolytic and osteosclerotic lesions on X-ray.
• Isotope bone scanning identifies affected bones but cannot differentiate Paget's disease from other bone disorders, e.g. metastatic disease (Figures 1.60 and 1.61).

 • Pathological fracture.
• Spinal stenosis and paraplegia.
• Osteoarthritis.
• Diplopia.
• Deafness.
• High-output cardiac failure.
• Malignant change to osteosarcoma (rare – 1%).

 • Initial osteolytic stage.
• Followed by a mixed osteolytic–osteoblastic stage that evolves ultimately into ...
• A burnt-out quiescent osteosclerotic stage.

 Treat complications medically with calcitonin and bisphosphonates.

Median nerve injury

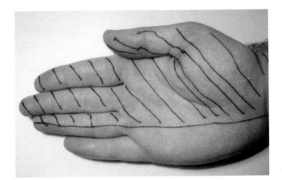

Figure 1.62

On clinical examination, a 24-year-old male who had received a stab injury to the anterior aspect of the distal aspect of the right forearm had the sensory loss demonstrated.

Questions

Q1 Which nerve has been injured?

Q2 What muscles does this nerve supply in the hand? Describe how you would test this clinically.

Q3 How would the sensory loss described above differ in the case of carpal tunnel syndrome?

Q4 Name two clinical tests for carpal tunnel syndrome.

Q5 Name some conditions associated with carpal tunnel syndrome.

Answers

A1 The median nerve. Note that clinically, the sensory loss is most easily detected over the pulps of the index and middle fingers.

A2 It supplies:
- the lateral two **L**umbricals
- the **O**pponens pollicis
- the **A**bductor pollicis brevis
- the **F**lexor pollicis brevis in the hand.

(Mnemonic: LOAF)

The best test is to test abductor pollicis brevis by abducting the thumb, at right angles to the palm, against resistance.

A3 There should be no paraesthesiae or loss of sensation over the thenar eminence as this area of skin is supplied by the palmar cutaneous branch of the median nerve which arises proximal to the carpal tunnel.

A4
- Phalen's test: maximal flexion of the wrist for one minute producing symptoms.
- Tinel's sign: percussion of the nerve at the wrist causing paraesthesia.

A5
- Rheumatoid arthritis.
- Acromegaly.
- Hypothyroidism.
- Amyloid.
- Pregnancy.

Femoral neck fractures and avascular necrosis

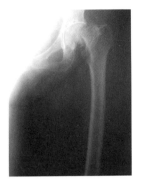

Figure 1.63

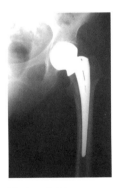

Figure 1.64

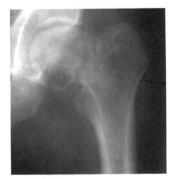

Figure 1.65

An 80-year-old lady slipped in the street and fell over onto her left side. She was unable to get up. In the accident and emergency department the

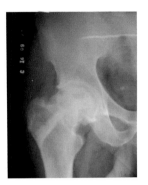

Figure 1.66

senior house officer astutely noticed that her left leg was shortened and externally rotated compared to the other side. He requested a plain film of her pelvis.

Questions

Q1 What is the diagnosis (Figure 1.63)? What other view should he have also requested?

Q2 How do you classify this condition and how does this relate to management? What has this patient had done (Figure 1.64)?

Q3 What are the possible complications? What do Figures 1.65 and 1.66 show?

Q4 What is the blood supply to the femoral head?

Q5 When is this an orthopaedic emergency?

Q6 What are the prognosis and possible complications of surgery?

Q7 What surgical approaches to the hip do you know of? Which nerves are at risk?

Answers

 • Left intracapsular neck of femur fracture.
 • He should have requested a lateral view too, to assess displacement.

 Neck of femur fractures are broadly divided into **intracapsular** and **extracapsular** fractures.
Intracapsular fractures
These include subcapital, cervical and basi-cervical fractures: they tend to disrupt the blood supply to the femoral head (see above). There is an increased risk of avascular necrosis of the head.

Garden classification for intracapsular fractures
This describes the degree of displacement at the fracture site:
• *Type I*: incomplete fracture
• *Type II*: complete but undisplaced fracture
• *Type III*: complete fracture with partial displacement
• *Type IV*: complete fracture with complete displacement.
The type of fracture dictates surgical management:
• *undisplaced intracapsular fractures*: internal fixation with 2–3 cannulated parallel screws
• *displaced intracapsular fractures*: hemiarthroplasty in the elderly, e.g. simple unipolar prosthesis Austin Moor or Thompson; fit patients <65 years should be treated by reduction and internal fixation or consideration for bipolar hemiarthroplasty.

Extracapsular fractures
These include intertrochanteric, basal and sub-trochanteric fractures and are distal to the insertion of the capsule. Classification is based on the number of fragments produced by the fracture:
• *undisplaced* (two-part)
• *displaced* (two-part)
• *three-part* involving the greater trochanter
• *three-part* involving the lesser trochanter
• *four-part*
• *reverse oblique.*
Management depends on site and number parts of fracture:
• *intertrochanteric and basal fractures*: dynamic hip screw
• *sub-trochanteric fractures with open reduction*: internal fixation with intramedullary hip screw (IMHS).

This patient has had a left hemiarthroplasty (Austin Moor) performed.

 Complications of femoral neck fractures are:
• avascular necrosis (AVN): high risk in displaced fractures due to disruption of the blood supply. Eventually the femoral head collapses causing pain and loss of function
• non-union
• osteoarthritis
• non-specific: deep vein thrombosis, pulmonary embolism, chest infection, pressure sores.
Figure 1.65 shows AVN of the left femoral head; Figure 1.66 shows AVN of the right femoral head with fibular grafting.

(A4) There are **three** sources for the blood supply to the femoral head:
- through the diaphysis
- retinacular branches from the medial and lateral femoral circumflex arteries (trochanteric anastomosis), which pass proximally within the joint capsule to anastomose at the junction of the neck and articular surface
- artery in the ligamentum teres: negligible in adults but essential in children, when the femoral head is separated from the neck by the cartilage of the epiphyseal line.

(A5)
- The benefit of preserving the femoral head in younger adults is much greater, thus biologically young patients with displaced intracapsular fractures are rushed into theatre for open reduction and fixation.
- If there is no evidence for this, a wait of 48 h will not prejudice the outcome of hip fracture surgery.

(A6)
- Complications normally occur in the elderly, with a high number of co-morbid factors. The highest mortality risk occurs within 6 months – ~50%.
- The main complications are: infection, dislocation, femoral stem loosening and acetabular erosion.

(A7)
- *Anterior approach*: between the tensor fascia lata and sartorius. Then divide the rectus femoris and anterior third of the gluteus medius.
- *Lateral approach*: this involves splitting the tensor fascia lata, gluteus medius and minimus or detaching them from the greater trochanter. The superior gluteal nerve is at risk here.
- *Posterior approach*: skin incision is centred on the posterior part of the greater trochanter. Proximally it is curved towards the posterior superior iliac spine. After subcutaneous tissue, this involves splitting the gluteus maximus and detaching the piriformis, obturator internus and gemelli from the femur. This gets access to the posterior capsule of the hip joint. The sciatic nerve is at risk here.

Your revision notes:

Perthes' disease

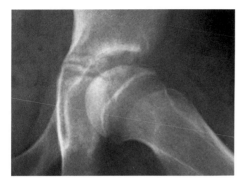

Figure 1.67

This 6-year-old boy limps into your outpatient clinic. Initially intermittent, the limp has become continuous over the past 2 months. This is the plain radiograph of his left hip.

Questions

Q1 What is the diagnosis?

Q2 What are the typical radiological features?

Q3 What groups of children are at risk of developing this condition?

Q4 What is the prognosis?

Q5 What is the management plan?

Answers

 The diagnosis is Perthes' disease. This condition is a self-limiting osteonecrosis of the femoral head that usually affects children aged between 4 and 8 years. M:F = 4:1.

 Radiographic appearance will depend upon the phase and extent of the disease. Usually there is an increase in joint space, flattening and increase in density of the femoral head.

 Groups at risk include those who:
- had low birth weight
- have a delayed bone age
- have a family history of the condition
- are from social classes 4 and 5.

- Also 1% of patients who get transient synovitis develop Perthes' disease.
- The cause is unknown.

 • The extent of disease is the most important prognostic factor.
- There are several classifications, which all depend on the amount of head affected. The more of the head affected the worse the prognosis. Generally if less than half of the head is affected the prognosis is good.

 • Rest and restriction of physical activity are required to relieve pain.
- Physiotherapy is required to maintain movement.
- Containment of the femoral head within the acetabulum avoids formation of a flattened irregular head and allows a more spherical head to develop; therefore a more congruous joint will decrease the risk of degenerative arthritis in the future. This can be achieved by maintaining movement, femoral osteotomies or plaster-cast bracing.

Scaphoid fracture

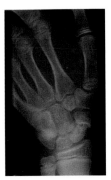

Figure 1.68

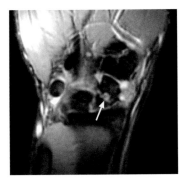

Figure 1.69

The radiograph in Figure 1.68 is taken from a 39-year-old male who fell on his outstretched hand.

Questions

Q1 What injury has he sustained?

Q2 Is this type of injury usually apparent on the initial X-ray? How can you accentuate the injury with imaging?

Q3 Is this injury more common in older people? What is the usual mechanism of injury?

Q4 What are the clinical signs?

Q5 What are the potential complications? What is the anatomical basis for them?

Q6 What is the management?

Q7 Look at Figure 1.69 (MRI scan), which was taken on another person with the same suspected injury. Why do you think this scan was organised?

Answers

(A1) Fracture through the waist of the scaphoid bone.

(A2) The fracture is not usually apparent on the initial X-ray. Request cards should be clearly marked as 'scaphoid' to ensure that at least **three** views of the scaphoid are obtained. 'Carpal box' views usually help in that they show the scaphoid elongated and magnified. The fracture gap can be maximised on imaging the wrist in ulnar deviation.

(A3) Scaphoid fractures often result from 'kickback' when using engine starter handles, or from falls onto the outstretched hand. They typically occur in young males and are not the most commonly seen fracture in older people.

(A4) Suspect a scaphoid fracture with the above-mentioned history:
- pain on the lateral aspect of the wrist usually with apparent tenderness in the anatomical snuffbox, although this is also a feature of many wrist sprains. In a true scaphoid fracture, tenderness will be found over the dorsal and palmar aspects of the scaphoid
- there may be marked swelling of the hand and wrist.

(A5)
- The most feared complication is avascular necrosis of the proximal segment of bone. The blood enters the scaphoid in a distal to proximal direction, and any fracture through the proximal segment is likely to lead to vascular disruption. Onset is usually immediate but a couple of months may elapse before the radiographs betray the presence of increased bone density. This leads to progressive bone collapse and radio-carpal osteoarthritis, leading to worsening stiffness and pain in the wrist.
- Non-union.
- Advanced osteoarthritis: usually a sequel to avascular necrosis or non-union.
- Sudeck's atrophy: a condition with unknown aetiology, which is essentially one of chronic post-traumatic pain with autonomic changes. There is swelling of the hand and fingers, which look pink with a glazed appearance and feel warm. This leads to movement restriction and diffuse pain in the wrist.

(A6)
- Undisplaced fractures (<2 mm) are treated in a plaster cast (scaphoid plaster) and sling for six weeks.
- The position of the hand is of importance: wrists should be fully pronated, radially deviated and moderately dorsiflexed.
- However some claim superior results with insertion of a Herbert screw with displaced fractures more than 1mm!
- The patient is reviewed at two weeks, and if the plaster is unduly slack this should be changed.
- The cast is removed at six weeks and if there is persistent tenderness at the fracture site the cast is reapplied for a further six weeks and then further radiographs are obtained.
- Continued signs of bone non-union are treated with bone grafting and Herbert compression screw insertion.
- Displaced fractures are treated initially with open reduction and insertion of a Herbert compression screw.

(A7) MRI shows a T_2-weighted MR image of the wrist. It shows a likely scaphoid fracture with bone oedema. Scaphoid fractures can sometimes be very difficult to identify on the radiographs despite three views being ordered. Repeat radiographs may have been inconclusive and therefore further imaging would have been obtained, usually in the form of an isotope bone scan or MRI (above). However all suspected scaphoid fractures should be treated on clinical grounds even if the radiographs are normal. The patient is usually re-imaged at 14 days, when local decalcification may reveal a previously hidden fracture.

Section 2

Critical care and trauma

Trauma

Abdominal trauma

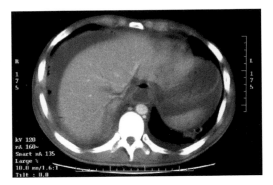

Figure 2.1

A 36-year-old male was brought into casualty with history of jumping out of a first-floor window. On arrival his GCS was 15/15, blood pressure 90/60 mmHg, pulse rate 100/min. Primary survey was performed and the patient was stabilised. Chest X-ray was normal. On secondary survey bruising was noted over the left lateral chest wall, with minimal tenderness over the lower ribs. Abdominal examination revealed generalised tenderness with minimal guarding in the epigastric and left upper quadrant regions. A CT scan of the abdomen was organised and is shown in Figure 2.1.

Questions

Q1 Describe the findings on the CT scan.

Q2 What is the most likely diagnosis and what is your reasoning?

Q3 How would you manage this condition?

Q4 What are the surgical options?

Answers

 The CT scan shows free fluid in the abdomen with blood surrounding the spleen.

 Splenic injury. The reasons for this diagnosis are:
- the low blood pressure on arrival
- bruising noted over the left lower chest wall
- left upper quadrant tenderness
- fluid collection around the spleen.

The clinical picture of splenic injury includes left upper quadrant pain and tenderness, signs of blood loss (low blood pressure, tachycardia, and features of shock) and pain in the left shoulder (Kehr's sign). Clinical signs can be surprisingly few. The injury mechanism should arouse suspicion.

Splenic injuries are associated with rib fractures, however lower ribs fractures can be missed on primary survey chest X-ray. Big splenic tears can be easily shown on CT.

 According to ATLS guidelines and emergency protocol:
- secure airway, breathing and circulation (ABC)
- two large-bore intravenous cannulas preferably in the antecubital fossa
- bloods for FBC, U&E, LFT, amylase, clotting profile and group and save. Cross-match 4–6 units of blood
- iv fluids: should be colloids
- primary and secondary surveys should be performed to rule out any other major injuries and also rule out any other source of shock
- if the patient is unstable and intra-abdominal pathology is suspected, he would need an emergency laparotomy
- if unsure of the diagnosis and if the patient is stable, he would need imaging such as a CT scan.

Rarely patients can present 12–24 h after injury, and if stable with a splenic injury, these patients can be treated conservatively, however, sequential CT scans may be needed. Delayed rupture can be seen as late as 2 weeks after injury in the non-operative group.

 Midline laparotomy is performed to evaluate the spleen for haemorrhage. Traditionally splenic injuries were always treated with splenectomy, now there has been a change in trend towards splenic salvage. In the first instance the spleen is mobilised and delivered into the abdominal wound to assess the splenic injury.
- Small capsular tears can be controlled with topical haemostatic agents.
- Lacerations into the splenic substance can be controlled with interlocking sutures.
- Major lacerations which involve more than 50% of splenic tissue can be treated with segmental splenic resection.
- If there is massive damage to the spleen, hilar injury, shattered spleen, or the patient is unstable with uncontrolled bleeding splenectomy is the best option.
- Other organs should be evaluated for simultaneous injury.

Black eye

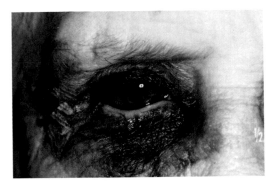

Figure 2.2

Questions

Q1 Describe what is shown in Figure 2.2.

Q2 What are the common mechanisms of injury?

Q3 What are the common causes of swellings around the eye?

Q4 How would you tailor your examination? What are the important things to elicit?

Q5 What are the treatment principles?

Answers

(A1) Common terminology describes it as 'black eye'; a peri-orbital black discoloration is seen with an extensive subconjunctival haemorrhage. There is evidence of minimal subconjunctival chemosis/oedema. The pupil margins are regular. There is a small laceration on the lateral aspect of the orbit, which has been steri-stripped.

(A2) The most common elicitable history is a 'punch' with a fist injury, e.g. mugging. In rare instances, an accidental cause such as a fall is possible. It can also occur in a road traffic accident, e.g. front seat passenger not wearing a seat belt.

(A3)
- Surgical procedures to the face, such as a facelift, jaw surgery, or nose surgery, can cause black eyes as well.
- A certain type of head injury, called a basilar skull fracture, causes both eyes to swell and blacken. This condition is typically described as 'raccoon's eyes' or 'panda eyes'.
- Other causes of swelling around the eye include allergic reactions, bites, cellulitis (skin infection around the eye), angioedema (hereditary condition causing swelling, usually around both eyes), and dental infections. However, these conditions do not make the skin turn black and blue around the eye.

(A4)
- Visual acuity measurement is very important medico-legally.
- Intra-orbital injury: can vary from a minor to major scale. This includes lacerations of the cornea/conjunctiva with subconjunctival haemorrhage. Avulsions of the iris leading to irregular pupil margins, retinal detachments, retinal oedema, and lens dislocations are possible. In certain circumstances there is a risk of intra-ocular foreign body implantation depending upon the offending object used to inflict the injury.
- Orbital blow out fracture can occur, in which the inferior plate of the orbit is injured as it is the weakest boundary. This can cause entrapment of the inferior oblique muscle or injury to the abducent nerve leading to diplopia.
- Other rims of the orbital plate can also be fractured if a significant force has been used. Associated nasal injuries are common including epistaxis, nasal bone fractures, septal haematoma and deviated nasal septum.
- X-rays confirm the fractures of the specific sites of the orbital rim. There is also an obliteration of the maxillary air sinus due to accumulation of blood or fluid exudation into the sinus.

(A5)
- Orbital injury will need urgent referral to an ophthalmologist, maxillofacial, plastic or ENT surgeon depending on the relevant scenario. Minor lacerations may only need suturing or steri-strips. Subconjunctival haemorrhage needs no active treatment, as spontaneous resolution is likely. Associated injury to the iris/cornea may need cycloplegics and prophylactic antibiotics, which are best dealt with by referral to the ophthalmologist.
- Intra-orbital injuries are similarly referred to the ophthalmologist. More severe injuries due to blunt trauma may be masked behind a superficial black eye. Hence, all cases of closed globe injuries should be referred to an ophthalmologist for confirming diagnosis and further management. An exploration should be carried out to release the muscle/nerve or both, and fixation of the blow out fracture as appropriate – this is best dealt with by referral to a maxillofacial surgeon. Nasal injuries are best dealt with by referral to an ENT surgeon and complicated lacerations of the face similarly referred to a plastic surgeon for reconstruction.

Hand injury

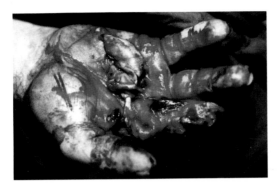

Figure 2.3

Questions

Q1 How do you classify hand injuries?

Q2 What are the principles of management of this type of injury?

Q3 What are the zones of the hand and what is their importance in reconstruction?

Q4 What is the order of repair in multiple flexor tendon injury at the wrist (Zone 5)?

Q5 What are the principles of tendon reconstruction?

Q6 What are the options available to repair tendon damage?

Q7 Classify nerve injuries.

Q8 What are the principles of nerve reconstruction?

Q9 What are the indications for replantation?

Q10 What are the basic surgical techniques employed during replantation?

Q11 What are the contraindications to replantation?

Q12 What are the potential complications? What are the options available to treat the complications?

Answers

 Tidy, **untidy** and **indeterminate**.

- To be assessed or treated under general anaesthetic if possible.
- Adequate analgesia.
- Tetanus prophylaxis.
- Prophylactic antibiotics.
- Thorough cleaning of the wounds and removal of debris, grit, dirt and grease. Debridement as appropriate.
- Hand dominance of the individual is significant in reconstruction.
- Incisions on the hand: Z-shaped when it overlies a joint/transverse limb; the Z shape incisions can overlie joint regions. Longitudinal incisions should only be made on the lateral aspects of the fingers.
- Failed primary repair is worse than no repair! If only one tendon is cut the functional result will be better than a poor repair.
- Adequate skin cover to keep exposure of the underlying tendons or bones to a minimum.
- The thumb receives the maximum priority at preservation as it has the maximum efficiency of the functioning hand. The index and the middle fingers are next in order of importance followed by the ring finger. The little finger is the least important.
- The amputated region is gently washed in Hartmann's solution wrapped in a swab, and should be preserved in a plastic bag surrounded by ice in a carrying container when it is transported to a specialist centre.
- Amputations are classified on the anatomical site. Mechanisms of amputation have a bearing on the outcome. They can be guillotined, crushed or avulsed. Avulsions have the poorest results and prognosis.
- Early post-operative intensive physiotherapy should be carried out to prevent contractures and disuse atrophy. Occupational rehabilitation may be needed in certain instances.
- Contraindications to repair include wounds liable to infection.

A3 The flexor tendons of the hand have attachments to the bony framework to avoid a bow stringing effect by a mechanism of pulleys:
- A1 pulley overlapping the flexor tendon sheath at the distal end of the metacarpals
- A2 pulley overlapping the flexor tendon sheath at the base of the proximal phalanx
- A3 pulley overlapping the flexor tendon sheath at the distal end of the proximal phalanx
- A4 pulley overlapping the flexor tendon sheath around the middle phalanx.

The hand is classified into five zones:
- Zone 1: FDP insertion to FDS insertion
- Zone 2: Zone 1 to proximal part of the A1 pulley
- Zone 3: zone 2 to distal edge of flexor retinaculum
- Zone 4: within the carpal tunnel
- Zone 5: proximal to the carpal tunnel.

 The order of repair is:
1 FPL
2 FDP tendons
3 FDS to middle and ring fingers
4 FDS to index and little fingers
5 ulnar nerve
6 ulnar artery

7 median nerve
8 FCU
9 FCR
10 radial artery – ligated.

A5
- Tendon reconstruction is done either as a primary repair or a delayed repair (after 3 weeks).
- Satisfactory dissection of the area is carried out to clearly identify and display both the proximal and distal ends of the severed tendon prior to anastomosis. Retracted tendons may have to be milked through or separate incisions may be needed.
- Use core non-absorbable 4/0 suture: modified Kessler technique.
- Use 6/0 monofilament running epitenon suture.
- Close the tendon sheath if possible.
- Badly damaged segment may need excision and sufficient mobilisation to attain a no-tension repair.

A6
- Primary or delayed direct repair.
- Single-stage flexor tendon grafting.
- Two-stage grafting.
- Tenodesis or arthrodesis.
- Tendon transfer.
- Amputation.

A7 **Seddon's classification**
- *Neurapraxia* is a reduction or complete block of conduction across a segment of a nerve, with axonal continuity conserved.
- *Axonotmesis* is a result of damage to the axons with preservation of the neural connective tissue sheath (endoneurium), epineurium, Schwann cell tubes, and other supporting structures. Thus, the internal architecture is relatively preserved. This can guide proximal axonal regeneration to reinnervate distal target organs. Distal Wallerian degeneration occurs in axonotmesis.
- *Neurotmesis* is the most severe grade of peripheral nerve injury. It occurs when the axon, myelin, and connective tissue components are damaged and disrupted or transected. This grade of injury includes nerve lesions in which external continuity is preserved but intraneural fibrosis occurs and blocks axonal regeneration.

Sunderland's classification
Sunderland categorised nerve injuries into five grades.
- *Grade I*: Seddon's neuropraxia.
- *Grade II*: Seddon's axonotmesis.
- *Grade III*: axon continuity is disrupted by loss of endoneurial tubes (the neurolemmal sheaths) but the perineurium is preserved. Thus, when the axons regenerate, they may enter an incorrect nerve sheath, resulting in abnormal regeneration.
- *Grade IV*: nerve fasciculi (i.e. axon, endoneurium, perineurium) are damaged but nerve sheath continuity is preserved.
- *Grade V*: the endoneurium, perineurium, and epineurium, which make up the entire nerve trunk, are completely divided.

A8
- Surgical intervention for acute nerve injury is based on the extent of damage to the nerve and the nerve's functional viability.
- In clean lacerating injuries in which the nerve ends are visible in the wound or when clinical examination reveals obvious motor and sensory deficits resulting from the injury at the laceration, immediate primary repair may be indicated but blunt transection due to lacerations has better results when done as a delayed surgical procedure.

- Accurate grading is necessary for identifying high-grade injuries that may benefit from early surgery, and for preventing unnecessary early exploration of grade I and II lesions.
- If nerve function is progressively deteriorating as shown by electrodiagnostic study findings, surgery may be indicated because the status of the connective tissue cannot be assessed without direct exploration.
- Routine electrodiagnostic testing can be used to support a clinical suspicion of nerve injury, or to evaluate the nerve function in patients in whom a reliable neurological examination is impossible.
- Contraindications to surgery usually result when the risks of surgery outweigh the benefits. Surgery should not be performed when a poor outcome is expected.
- In an epineurial repair, the epineuriums of the separated nerve endings are sutured together using a microsuture (usually 8-0 or 10-0 suture) with no tension at the anastomosis.
- The best results occur when the nerves are either purely sensory or purely motor, and when the intraneural connective tissue component is small and the fascicles have been clearly aligned.
- Excessive sutures add to scar tissue production. Individual fascicle repair is not practised because it requires numerous sutures and because it is technically difficult.
- Secondary repairs are delayed repairs that may entail different strategies like bone shortening or nerve transposition across a flexed joint, which can be done to add length to a nerve.
- Neurolysis is performed on intraneural and extraneural scar tissue to release regenerating nerve fibres in the hope of improving functional recovery.
- Many surgeons prefer delayed suture to primary suture because this allows the wound to heal and it decreases the risk of infection. In addition, during a delayed repair, scarred ends of the nerve can be defined more accurately and trimmed back to normal fasciculi. The epineurial suture is more secure because the sheath has toughened. The suture of a severed nerve should not be delayed beyond 1 month.
- Contaminated wounds, such as gunshot wounds and avulsions with severe tissue disruption, benefit from a secondary repair. Severely damaged nerves may require a nerve graft.
- Nerve or tendon transfers may be necessary for unrestorable or unsuccessful nerve repair.

- Thumb amputation.
- Multiple digit amputations.
- Metacarpal amputation.
- Almost any body part in a child.
- Wrist or forearm amputation.
- Individual digit distal to FDS insertion; replantation at a level distal to insertion of the FDS often results in satisfactory function.

Surgical technique, in sequence, is as follows:

1 bilateral mid-lateral incisions
2 isolate vessels and nerves and debridement as necessary
3 shorten and fix bone
4 repair the flexor and extensor tendons (in the case of a hand replantation the flexor and extensor tendons are repaired after arterial and venous flow has been established)
5 repair nerves (before arteries, since a tourniquet is required)

6 anastomosis of arteries (hand or forearm replantation, consider use of arterial shunt before the vascular anastomosis; give systemic heparin)
7 anastomosis of veins (two for each artery, or three veins minimum); veins are never repaired before arteries, especially in hand or forearm replants, since reperfusion toxins will enter into the body
8 skin coverage.

Local contraindications
- Severely crushed or mangled parts.
- Amputations at multiple levels.
- Distal amputations, amputations distal to the DIP joint are difficult to replant since the digital artery begins to branch and dorsal veins are hard to find.

General contraindications
- Amputations in patients with other serious injuries or diseases.
- Atherosclerotic vessels.
- Mentally unstable patients.

Early complications
- Arterial insufficiency:
  - inspect and loosen dressing
  - change hand position
  - stiletto block (spasm)
  - heparin bolus (3000 to 5000 units)
  - if no improvement in 4–6 h, return to theatre to re-do anastomosis: 50–60% successful.
- Venous insufficiency.

Late complications
- Functional difficulties:
  - related to 'one wound, one scar' concept with resultant loss of differential gliding between the tissues
  - motion of digits significantly affected by overall injury sustained, motion of the PIPJ accounts for 85% of the arc of finger motion.
- Cold intolerance:
  - thought to improve after 2 years but a recent long-term study has shown no improvement.

Nerve recovery
- Dependent on the type and level of injury, but overall the results are comparable to isolated nerve injuries.
- Two-point discrimination: adults 11 mm, children 9 mm.
- Fine tactile discrimination rarely returns.

Your revision notes:

Pelvic injury

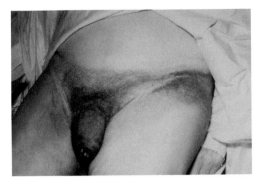

Figure 2.4

Questions

Q1 What is shown in Figure 2.4?

Q2 Classify pelvic fractures.

Q3 What are the signs of a pelvic injury?

Q4 How is the situation managed?

Answers

Bruising around the groins and the perineum and a possible urethral injury secondary to a pelvic fracture.

- *Minor pelvic fracture*: varies from an isolated chip in the pelvic brim to single cracks and undisplaced pubic rami fracture.
- *Major pelvic fracture*:
  - *anterior–posterior fracture*: AP compression injury leading to pubic rami fracture with displacement leading to associated bladder or urethral injury
  - *vertical displacement fracture*: resulting from fall from heights producing vertical displacement of the hemi-pelvis and associated injury to the sciatic nerve or pelvic viscera
  - *open book fracture*: the pelvis is opened out and there is sacroiliac diastasis with a massive retro-pelvic haemorrhage
  - *combined displacement*: when there is a combination of the forces.
- *Acetabular fracture.*

- Bruising in the groins, around the iliac crests, the perineum and the external genitalia.
- Blood at the external urethral meatus.
- Tenderness on pelvic springing on the ATLS pelvis compression manoeuvre.
- Hypovolaemic shock due to the tearing of the pelvic veins in the event of major pelvic fractures disrupting the pelvic ring.
- Retention of urine: due to injury to the urethra – complete or partial avulsion of the junction of the prostatic and membranous urethra.
- Intraperitoneal rupture of the bladder with peritonitis.
- Extraperitoneal rupture of the bladder with extravasation of urine superficial to the scarpa's fascia in the perineum and the lower abdominal wall.
- High-riding prostate on a per rectal examination.
- Pelvic viscera injury (rectum/other bowels).
- Sciatic nerve injuries (neuropraxia and axontemesis are more common) with foot drop.

Resuscitation according to ATLS protocols with appropriate X-rays. MAST suits may be needed in the initial resuscitation period. Massive blood transfusions may be needed. A CT scan is helpful to assess pelvic injury after adequate resuscitation.

Pelvic injury
Minor injuries
- Conservative management with bed rest for 1–3 weeks on a soft mattress placed on a fracture board, followed by early mobilisation.

Major injuries
- Splinting the fracture helps significantly to minimise the blood loss from the pelvic veins and also in the control of pain. Stabilisation of the pelvis with external fixators may be necessary. Pelvic vein embolisation may be needed to control the haemorrhage. This is followed by a more definite pelvic fixation with plate and screws in a more appropriate centre after stabilising the patient.
- Open book-type of fractures may need to be nursed in the lateral position to close the fracture before stabilisation with fixators. The affected leg may be balanced on a canvas sling with traction if needed.
- If there is a minimal vertical displacement of the hemipelvis then skin traction to reduce it may be needed, followed by non-weight-bearing mobilisation after 6 weeks.

- If there is a severe vertical displacement of the hemipelvis then Steinmann pin traction applied through the tibial tuberosity or the lower end of femur may be needed. This is followed by non-weight-bearing mobilisation after 2–3 months.
- Acetabular injuries are treated with traction/conservative methods. Exploration may be necessary for complicated injuries.

Urethral injury
- Prophylactic antibiotics cover is necessary.
- An urgent ascending urethrogram to determine the site, extent and the length of the segment of the injury may be needed.
- An IVU may also be needed to evaluate the upper tracts.
- Alignment is facilitated by the stabilisation/fixation of the pelvic ring.
- Utmost care and gentle manoeuvres are compulsory for fear of converting a partial urethral injury to a complete one.
- If there is injury to the membranous urethra then gentle catheterisation with a soft catheter is needed. If this fails then exploration is needed. The bladder is opened and a urethral sound inserted through the prostatic urethra to facilitate a 'rail road' technique to establish the continuity in the injured urethra. Once the catheter is in place, it is left *in situ* for about 3 weeks.
- If there is extraperitoneal rupture of the bladder then a urethral catheter and a suprapubic drain may be needed. The catheter is left for 2 weeks to allow healing.
- If there is intraperitoneal rupture of the bladder then a laparotomy and two-layer closure with a urethral catheter for 2–3 weeks is needed. A suprapubic catheter may be placed if needed.
- Long-term complications include urethral strictures, which may need further procedures like dilatations or reconstructions.

Neuronal injury
Injuries to the sciatic nerve or the lumbosacral plexus are commonly neuropraxia or axontemesis and usually recover well with conservative management. However, the results are poor if there is neurotemesis. Exploration is needed if there is a bony spicule causing the possible nerve lesion.

Bowel injury
This may need urgent laparotomy and repair with or without a diversion stoma. Paralytic ileus is common after pelvic injuries.

Your revision notes:

Critical care

Hypoxia

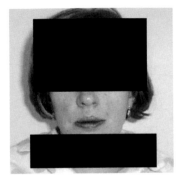

Figure 2.5

This 54-year-old patient had a hemicolectomy two days ago after bowel perforation due to diverticulitis. She complains of shortness of breath. On examination she is cyanosed, tachypnoeic, with bilateral fine crackles and decreased air entry in the lung bases. Arterial blood gas analysis (on room air) shows the following:

pH	7.36
$Paco_2$	4.1 kPa
Pao_2	6.2 kPa

Questions

Q1 What is the diagnosis?

Q2 What is the problem with this patient's arterial blood gas?

Q3 How would you classify it?

Q4 What do you think is the cause in this case?

Q5 How would you initiate treatment?

Q6 A diagnosis of ARDS is made and the above measures are not successful. What other measures are to be considered?

Q7 Despite all of the above (on 100% O_2, PEEP 15 kPa, prone protective ventilation strategy), the patient still has a Pao_2 of 7.1 kPa only, with $Paco_2$ 8.9 kPa. Is there anything else that can be done?

Answers

(A1) Central cyanosis.

(A2) Hypoxia.

(A3) **Hypoxic hypoxia**
This is a reduction in the amount of oxygen passing into the blood, due to one of the following:
- alveolar ventilation–perfusion mismatch
- diffusion impairment
- venous-to-arterial shunts (between vessels or within the heart)
- reduced atmospheric pressure.

Anaemic hypoxia (reduced oxygen-binding capacity of blood)
- Low haemoglobin levels.
- Met-haemoglobinaemia.
- CO-haemoglobinaemia.

Histotoxic hypoxia (insufficient oxygen extraction in tissues)
- e.g. Cyanide poisoning (mitochondrial block).

Stagnant hypoxia
- Malfunction of the circulatory system, which reduces generalised blood flow through tissues. While the oxygen-carrying capacity of the blood is adequate, there is an inadequate circulation of the blood.
- Conditions with arterial occlusion lead to localised tissue hypoxia.

(A4) The likely causes are atelectasis, pneumonia, lobar collapse, pulmonary embolism or acute respiratory distress syndrome (ARDS).

(A5)
- Increasing the FIO_2 could buy time to investigate the cause and make a firm diagnosis which may need specific treatment.
- Sitting the patient up, optimising analgesia and encouraging deep breaths and coughing may be all that is required if it is atelectasis only. Physiotherapy can be of help.

(A6)
- Continuous positive airway pressure (CPAP).
- Tracheal intubation with mechanical ventilation of some sort.
- Recruitment of alveoli with various techniques:
  - positive end-expiratory pressure (PEEP)
  - inverse ratio ventilation (longer inspiratory phase)
  - prone ventilation
  - recruitment manoeuvres (various options, e.g. prolonged PEEP of 30–40 s without any breaths to encourage expansion of so-called slow alveoli)
  - high-frequency ventilation.

(A7) Consider referral to an extracorporeal membrane oxygenation (ECMO) centre.

Acute respiratory distress syndrome

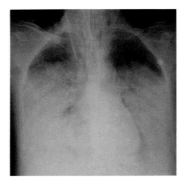

Figure 2.6

Questions

Q1 What is the most obvious diagnosis on this chest X-ray?

Q2 What are the causes and the underlying pathophysiology?

Q3 How does the patient with this condition present?

Q4 How is it diagnosed?

Q5 What is the treatment?

Answers

(A1) This is an intubated patient with evidence of ARDS and a pneumomediastinum.

(A2) • ARDS is a life-threatening medical emergency with patients becoming acutely hypoxic. The mortality rate is approximately 40–50%. Various acute processes that directly or indirectly injure the lung can cause it. Sepsis is often encountered as a cause, as are pneumonia, aspiration of gastric contents, prolonged or profound shock, lung contusion, burns, fat embolism, near drowning, massive blood transfusion, acute haemorrhagic pancreatitis and inhalation of smoke or other toxic gas.
   • Apparently activated white blood cells and platelets accumulate in capillaries, the interstitium, and airspaces of the lung. They may release prostaglandins, free radicals, enzymes, tumour necrosis factor and interleukins. Pulmonary capillary and alveolar epithelia are injured, and plasma and blood leak into the interstitial and intra-alveolar spaces. Atelectasis results partly due to reduced surfactant activity. The injury is not homogeneous and affects mainly the dependent lung zones.
   • Within 2 to 3 days, interstitial and broncho-alveolar inflammation develop, and epithelial and interstitial cells proliferate. Then, collagen may accumulate rapidly, resulting in severe interstitial fibrosis within 2 to 3 weeks. These pathological changes lead to low lung compliance, decreased functional residual capacity, ventilation/perfusion imbalances, increased physiological dead space, severe hypoxaemia, and pulmonary hypertension.

(A3) Onset of symptoms is usually within 24–48 h after the initial insult. Dyspnoea occurs first, usually accompanied by rapid, shallow respiration and cyanosis. Auscultation may detect crackles, rhonchi, or wheezes, or findings may be normal. The primary cause may be obvious or concealed.

(A4) Early diagnosis requires a high index of suspicion. A presumptive diagnosis can be made with arterial blood gas analysis and chest X-rays. Chest X-rays usually show diffuse bilateral alveolar infiltrates similar to acute pulmonary oedema of cardiac origin, but the cardiac silhouette is usually normal. However, the severity of changes seen on X-ray often lags many hours behind functional changes. The extremely low PaO_2 often persists despite high concentrations of inspired O_2 (FIO_2), indicating pulmonary right-to-left shunting through atelectatic and consolidated lung units that are not ventilated. Cardiogenic pulmonary oedema needs to be excluded by definition, i.e. pulmonary capillary wedge pressure (PCWP) low (<18 mmHg) in ARDS and high (>20 mmHg) in heart failure. The current swing away from Swan–Ganz catheters necessitates other ways to rule out cardiac failure. Echocardiography is very useful in that respect. Pulmonary embolism, which may mimic ARDS, may need to be ruled out by pulmonary angiography. Lung biopsy or bronchoscopy may be needed to rule out other pulmonary conditions.

(A5) • Despite different aetiologies, the management principles are similar. General supportive treatment is essential. While the diagnosis is being considered, life-threatening hypoxaemia must be treated with a high FIO_2 and monitored with repeated arterial blood gases or non-invasive oximetry. Prompt endotracheal intubation with mechanical ventilation and PEEP may be needed to deliver O_2 because hypoxaemia is frequently refractory to O_2 inhalation by face-mask.
   • The underlying cause of acute lung injury needs to be corrected. Re-exploration of the abdomen should be considered where the potential for abdominal sepsis exists. Meticulous attention is necessary to prevent nutritional depletion, O_2 toxicity, superinfection, barotrauma, and renal failure, which may be worsened by intravascular volume depletion.

- Conventional settings on a ventilator aim for a tidal volume of 10–15 ml/kg, a PEEP of 5–10 cmH$_2$O, and an Fio$_2$ of <0.6. There is concern that high ventilator pressures and volumes in ARDS can worsen lung injury. A PEEP that is too low can also damage the lung by allowing unstable terminal lung units to open and close repeatedly. This problem may be circumvented with small tidal volumes (6–8 ml/kg) and a higher PEEP (between 10 and 18 cmH$_2$O). The latter approach has become known as protective ventilation and is the accepted standard.
- Ventilator plateau pressure is measured, with the aim not to exceed 25–30 cmH$_2$O. With a reduced tidal volume, the respiratory rate of the ventilator can be increased to maintain an adequate arterial pH and Pco$_2$. Some patients still develop hypercapnia and respiratory acidosis, which are usually well tolerated.

Your revision notes:

Barotrauma

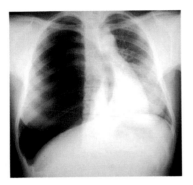

Figure 2.7

Questions

Q1 What is the diagnosis in this CXR?

Q2 What is the treatment?

Q3 What are the causes?

Q4 What are the iatrogenic causes?

Q5 How does ventilator-induced barotrauma occur?

Q6 What is the pathophysiology of tension pneumothorax?

Q7 Under what circumstances can high pressure in the lung be expected?

Q8 Is there any other mechanism by which injury can be inflicted by ventilation?

Answers

(A1) Tension pneumothorax.

(A2) If the patient's condition is stable, an urgent intercostal drain (ICD) is inserted. If unstable, a needle is inserted in the second intercostal space in the mid-clavicular line. Connecting the needle to a syringe with saline will show air under pressure bubbling in the saline. However if the pressure is high it will make an unmistakable hissing noise. An ICD should follow needle decompression.

(A3) Tension pneumothorax is most often related to trauma of some kind, e.g. a knife wound, fractured ribs or severe coughing in a patient with emphysematous bullae. It may occur during an acute asthma attack but can occur spontaneously, typically in tall thin individuals. Rapid ascent from a dive at depth leads to lung expansion and rupture if the glottis is kept closed. This was the first situation where pulmonary barotrauma was recognised.

(A4)
- Many types of surgery may be responsible and it is often obvious, but occasionally concealed, e.g. laparoscopic repair of hiatus hernia and nephrectomy.
- Direct trauma when inserting subclavian central lines (rarely with internal jugular lines).
- Brachial plexus blocks.
- Bronchoscopy.
- Double lumen tubes.
- Vigorous suctioning.
- Chest compression during CPR.
- Traumatic attempts at intubating the trachea or passing nasogastric tubes.
- Barotrauma while on a ventilator.

(A5) When a certain, often unpredictable, level of intrapulmonary pressure is reached, small tears will occur in the alveolar tissue. This may lead to air under pressure tracking in tissue planes to coalesce and rupture into the pleura. This is more likely to happen in certain conditions where high ventilation pressures tend to occur, or where the lung itself is pathologically stiff. This may lead to air accumulating in the pleura and eventually compressing the lung.

(A6)
- As the pressure increases, the ipsilateral lung collapses and causes hypoxia. Further pressure build-up causes the mediastinum to shift toward the contralateral side and impinge on both the contralateral lung and the vasculature entering the right atrium of the heart. This condition leads to worsening hypoxia and compromised venous return.
- Cardiovascular collapse develops from a combination of mechanical and hypoxic effects. The mechanical effects manifest as high intrathoracic pressure exceeding the low-pressure venous system. Obstruction of the superior and inferior vena cavae due to kinking or compression contributes. Mediastinal shift can cause a vaso-vagal attack. Hypoxia leads to increased pulmonary vascular resistance via vasoconstriction. Cardiac output decreases and metabolic acidosis results from decreased oxygen delivery to the periphery. If the underlying problem remains untreated, the hypoxia, metabolic acidosis, and decreased cardiac output lead to cardiac arrest and death.

- In patients with lung pathology which decreases compliance, e.g. pneumonia, ARDS.
- In conditions with airway obstruction, e.g. chronic obstructive airways disease (COPD), acute asthma attacks, auto-PEEP due to ventilator settings.
- Inappropriate ventilator settings.
- Hand-ventilation using a system without a pressure release valve.
- Endobronchial intubation.

Several studies have shown that ventilation with large tidal volumes results in an increased production of TNF-α and interleukin-6 in the systemic circulation. This may contribute to the development of a systemic inflammatory response syndrome and distal organ dysfunction.

Your revision notes:

Airway management

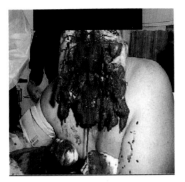

Figure 2.8

Questions

Q1 What are the obvious emergency problems that need to be addressed in this patient?

Q2 How can the circulatory volume be maintained?

Q3 How should the airway be maintained?

Q4 Before sedating or anaesthetising the patient, confirmation of the correct position of the endotracheal tube (ETT) is always essential. What is the most accurate method to confirm correct placement of the ETT?

Q5 If the airway is still not secured, a surgical airway will be the safest option. What is the next step?

Answers

(A1) Maintaining the airway and supporting the circulation.

(A2) Head and neck wounds tend to bleed profusely. Until surgical haemostasis can be secured, direct pressure on bleeding areas is essential. Avoiding venous engorgement by sitting up will also help. Good venous access for rapid replacement of blood loss will be essential. Recognisable bleeders need to be clamped.

(A3) • Spontaneous breathing will be essential and awake intubation ideal. Maintaining the upright sitting position, leaning slightly forward, will keep the airway open by forces of gravity. It is essential to maintain full consciousness until ready to secure an artificial airway for surgical purposes. Limit analgesia to the minimum to keep the patient comfortable without causing drowsiness. Avoid sedation or hypovolaemia which will lead to a tendency to fall back with loss of airway control.
  • While sitting, careful suctioning may demonstrate the tongue. This may be followed posteriorly by vision or palpation to find the epiglottis, which of course will make intubation easy. Another reason to ensure spontaneous breathing with minimal sedation is to allow the patient to cough or breathe rapidly to prevent aspiration of blood. It will also show bubbles or air movement to identify the larynx if it is obscured by blood or debris.

(A4) The only clinical sign that is accurate in more than 99% of cases is the ability to clearly see the ETT passing between the vocal cords. This is not even possible in many elective cases and in a trauma case with blood in the pharynx, it is extremely unlikely there will be a good view. End-tidal CO_2 detection, with a capnograph or disposable chemical detector, is the most useful ancillary device. This is of little diagnostic use in the cardiac arrest situation, when the oesophageal detector device is more useful. The latter is a device that creates a negative pressure when a syringe plunger is pulled out, or when a compressed rubber bulb is released. This negative pressure, when connected to an ETT in the oesophagus, leads to occlusion of the tube by the collapsible oesophagus. When connected to the ETT in the trachea, no collapse takes place and the bulb expands rapidly or the plunger can be pulled out with no resistance.

(A5) A crico-thyroidotomy under local anaesthesia, with the patient maintained in the sitting position, will be safest. Forcing the patient to lie down for a surgical tracheotomy will lead to airway obstruction and restlessness, and if sedation is added, disaster is imminent. Once crico-thyroidotomy is completed, the patient can be anaesthetised and intubated via the larynx to allow a formal surgical tracheotomy after haemostasis is obtained.

Sepsis

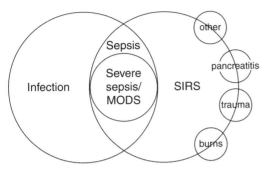

Sources:
Bone RC *et al. Chest.* 1992; **101**: 1644–55.
Vincent JL. *Crit Care Med.* 1997: **25**: 372–4.

Figure 2.9

Questions

Q1 The management of sepsis is an insignificant factor viewed in the perspective of total healthcare. True/False?

Q2 This famous diagram from 1992 indicates the link between these common and serious conditions. It is still very relevant today. What do you understand by the term systemic inflammatory response syndrome (SIRS)?

Q3 How does SIRS differ from sepsis?

Q4 Define severe sepsis.

Q5 What do you understand by the term septic shock?

Answers

 False. Sepsis represents a major health issue.
- Severe sepsis is associated with a mortality of almost 30% in the best centres.
- It is the cause of 215 000 deaths each year in the USA.
- Sepsis consumes a large part of the healthcare budget of most developed countries. The annual cost burden of severe sepsis is:
  - UK: approximately £0.25–0.29 billion
  - EU: approximately £4.1–5.4 billion
  - USA: approximately £11.3 billion.

 SIRS is a non-specific clinical response including two of the following:
- temperature >38°C or <36°C
- heart rate >90 beats/min
- respiratory rate >20/min
- white blood cell count >12 000/mm³ or <4000/mm³ or >10% immature neutrophils.

SIRS can be caused by infection, as well as trauma, burns, pancreatitis and other insults.

 Sepsis is equivalent to SIRS, but with a presumed or confirmed infectious origin.

(A4) Severe sepsis is sepsis with signs of at least one acute organ dysfunction, e.g.
- renal
- respiratory
- hepatic
- haematological
- central nervous system
- unexplained metabolic acidosis
- cardiovascular.

(A5) Septic shock is severe sepsis with hypotension, refractory to adequate volume resuscitation.

Sepsis management

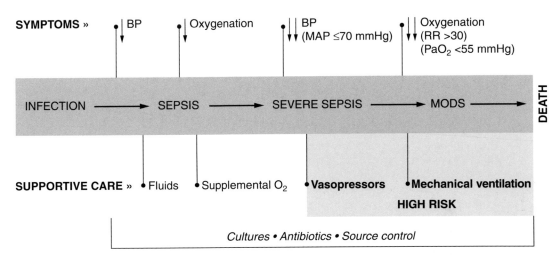

SYMPTOMS »

BP   Oxygenation   BP (MAP ≤70 mmHg)   Oxygenation (RR >30) (PaO₂ <55 mmHg)

INFECTION ⟶ SEPSIS ⟶ SEVERE SEPSIS ⟶ MODS ⟶ DEATH

SUPPORTIVE CARE »   • Fluids   • Supplemental O₂   • **Vasopressors**   • **Mechanical ventilation**

HIGH RISK

Cultures • Antibiotics • Source control

Figure 2.10

Questions

Q1 In addition to the management scheme outlined in Figure 2.10 by Michael P Keane MD, list additional modern measures to combat the results of sepsis.

Q2 Methyl prednisolone 30 mg/kg iv is essential in septic shock. True/False?

Q3 What are the side-effects of steroid therapy?

Q4 Is it possible to identify steroid responders in sepsis?

Q5 Are mineralocorticoids of any use in septic shock?

Q6 Do corticosteroids have any value in sepsis without shock?

Answers

 • Corticosteroids.
• Tight glucose control.
• Activated protein C.
• Protective ventilation strategies.
• Goal-directed therapy.

 False. Such large doses have been associated with major complications and increased death rate. Hydrocortisone 200–300 mg/day iv, for 7 days in three or four divided doses or by continuous infusion is recommended in patients with septic shock who, despite adequate fluid replacement, require inotropes or vasopressors to maintain adequate blood pressure. Dexamethasone 3 mg every 6 h has been recommended by some, as it does not interfere with cortisol measurement.

 The following adverse reactions have been reported with the systemic use of corticosteroids:
• *musculoskeletal*: steroid myopathy, muscle weakness, osteoporosis, pathological; fractures, vertebral compression fractures, aseptic necrosis of femoral and humeral heads, tendon rupture – particularly of the Achilles tendon
• *fluid and electrolyte disturbances*: sodium retention, fluid retention, hypertension, potassium loss, hypokalaemic alkalosis, diuresis, sodium excretion, congestive heart failure in susceptible patients
• *gastrointestinal*: peptic ulcer with possible perforation and haemorrhage, pancreatitis, oesophagitis, perforation of the bowel, transient nausea, vomiting or dysgeusia (with rapid administration of large doses)
• *hepatic*: increases in ALT, AST and alkaline phosphatase have been observed following corticosteroid treatment. These changes are usually small, not associated with any clinical syndrome and are reversible upon discontinuation
• *dermatological*: impaired wound healing, petechiae and ecchymoses, thin fragile skin
• *endocrine*: decreased carbohydrate tolerance, manifestations of latent diabetes mellitus, increased requirements for insulin or oral hypoglycaemic agents in diabetics, menstrual irregularities, development of Cushingoid state, suppression of the pituitary–adrenal axis, suppression of growth in children
• *metabolic*: negative nitrogen balance due to protein catabolism
• *neurological*: increased intracranial pressure, pseudotumour cerebri, psychic derangements, seizures
• *ophthalmic*: posterior subcapsular cataracts, increased intraocular pressure, exophthalmos
• *immunological*: masking of infections, latent infections becoming active, opportunistic infections, hypersensitivity reactions including anaphylaxis, may suppress reactions to skin tests.
The following additional reactions are related to parenteral corticosteroid therapy: anaphylactic reaction with or without circulatory collapse, cardiac arrest, bronchospasm, cardiac arrhythmias, hypotension or hypertension.

 The identification of relative adrenal insufficiency is based on:
• random cortisol level of <15 µg/dl (levels differ from lab to lab)
• a level between 15 and 34 µg/dl warrants a corticotrophin stimulation test
• when cortisol assays are not possible, empirical treatment is justified in selected cases.

(A5) Some experts would add fludrocortisone (50 mcg orally four times per day).

(A6) In the absence of shock, corticosteroids should not be administered for the treatment of sepsis.

Your revision notes:

Fluid balance

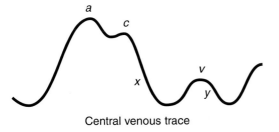

Central venous trace

Figure 2.11

Questions

Q1 Explain what happens physiologically during the various components of the central venous pressure trace (Figure 2.11).

Q2 How can the CVP be used in the haemodynamically unstable or oliguric patient?

Q3 What can be done to evaluate fluid balance if a central line is not present, not possible or contraindicated?

Q4 What is the preferred resuscitation fluid?

Answers

- The *a wave* is due to atrial contraction. It is absent in atrial fibrillation and enlarged in tricuspid stenosis, pulmonary stenosis and pulmonary hypertension.
- The *c wave* is due to bulging of the tricuspid valve into the right atrium, or possibly to transmitted pulsations from the carotid artery.
- The *x descent* is due to atrial relaxation.
- The *v wave* is due to the rise in atrial pressure before the tricuspid valve opens. It is enlarged in tricuspid regurgitation.
- The *y descent* is due to atrial emptying as blood enters the ventricle.
- *Canon waves* are large waves not corresponding to a, v or c waves. They are due to complete heart block or junctional arrhythmias.

There are various ways to use the CVP. A single target number is often aimed for, but least useful. The following example of a protocol for fluid loading has been found useful.

- This is not meant for the patient who is obviously hypovolaemic and needs large volumes of fluid or blood. This protocol is designed for all conditions where intravascular depletion is suspected but the degree is uncertain. This protocol need not be followed rigidly if the physician involved is with the patient or understands the patient's fluid needs and cardiovascular reserve.
- The physician must specify the type and volume of fluid required.
- The volume is specified in quantities of X, where $X = 50$, 100 or 200 ml, etc. The amount and type of fluid depend on the physician's assessment of the patient's risk of being overloaded, e.g. cardiovascular reserve, degree of fluid depletion, etc.
- Observe for 10 min:

CVP reading (mmHg)	Action
>12	X ml given iv
6–12	2 times X ml given iv
<6	3 times X ml given iv

If during infusion, >5 mmHg increase: STOP infusion, re-assess.

If following infusion, 2–5 mm Hg increase: wait 10 min, repeat if <2 mmHg increase.

If >2 mmHg increase: wait 20 min, re-assess.

If <2 mmHg increase: repeat entire challenge.

If >5 mmHg increase: STOP.

- Fluid administration is continued until haemodynamic signs of shock disappear, urine output improves or until the relevant rule is violated. If the possibility of fluid overload exists, e.g. falling oxygen saturation, sudden increase in respiratory rate or signs of dyspnoea occur, consider the use of an inotropic agent or diuretics.
- These parameters should be used in conjunction with clinical signs of hypovolaemia or hypervolaemia. In addition to the above, cardiac output studies and oxygen delivery studies may be done as well. Fluid challenges can also be given with heart rate, BP, urine output and other clinical signs alone used as endpoints but need a lot more caution.

(A3) Clinical signs as mentioned above are useful, as well as capillary refill time, skin turgor, dryness of oral mucosa and dampness of the axillae. Examining the jugular venous pulse in the neck is still useful in the fluid-overloaded patient. It is well known that femoral venous catheters can be used for CVP measurement. Less well known is the fact that peripheral venous cannulae can be used for CVP measurement. A prerequisite is a continuous fluid column between the transducer and the right atrium. It is imperative that the vein in the arm or leg should be unobstructed by external pressure or pathological masses. A good correlation with centrally measured CVP can be expected if coughing or breathing excursions are transmitted to the pressure curve. A peripheral measurement can be expected to be about 5–7 mmHg higher than a central measurement. In paediatric practice cannulae smaller than 20 g have not yet been validated.

(A4) There is no scientific evidence that synthetic colloids are any better or worse than crystalloids. Blood and blood products need to be replaced as indicated.

Your revision notes:

Starling curves

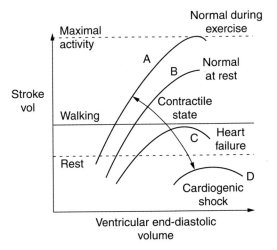

Figure 2.12

Questions

Q1 What is the use of the Frank–Starling curve to the clinician?

Q2 Is it safe to use CVP as an indicator of preload?

Q3 What determines venous return to the heart?

Q4 How do changes in inotropy affect the Starling curve?

The law of the heart is thus the same as the law of muscular tissue generally, that the energy of contraction, however measured, is a function of the length of the muscle fibre.

Answers

  • Otto Frank (late 19th century) and Ernest Starling (early 20th century) demonstrated that when the cardiac muscle becomes stretched an extra amount, as it does when extra amounts of blood enter the cardiac chambers, the stretched muscle contracts with a greatly increased force, thereby automatically pumping the extra blood into the arteries.
  • Preload or filling pressures (CVP and PCWP) are measured. That is a substitute for end-diastolic volume which again reflects the length of the stretched sarcomeres, which in turn respond by more forceful contraction.
  • This principle is used when patients are given fluid boluses to see how they respond. The clinician is (subconsciously) drawing a curve to find at which length of the sarcomere (actually which preload) the best stroke volume is delivered. Most often this is done without the ability to measure SV or CO, but the BP response is assessed as a simple substitute.

A2 Left ventricular end-diastolic pressure (reflected by the CVP or right atrial pressure) is occasionally an unreliable index of preload because the ventricular volume is determined by the compliance of the ventricle. Therefore, there can be an increase in end-diastolic pressure without an increase in preload due to a reduction in ventricular compliance, e.g. in ventricular hypertrophy and ischaemia. Furthermore when only a CVP is available, the interposing valves, lungs and heart need to be normal to be able to use the CVP as a substitute. This means that when fluid loading is given, the clinician needs to have an open mind to interpret the numbers. Careful loading is essential when it is uncertain on which curve the patient moves and where on the curve they belong. Single readings are of little value and the trend is important!

A3 Venous return is the flow of blood back to the heart, i.e. the preload. It is impeded by:
  • intravascular depletion
  • raised intrathoracic pressure seen in acute asthmatic attacks with auto-PEEP
  • tension pneumothorax
  • pericardial tamponade
  • constrictive pericarditis
  • mechanical ventilation, especially settings with high PEEP, inversed inspiratory: expiratory (I:E) ratios
  • inappropriate prone positioning with inferior vena cava compression
  • abdominal compartment syndrome.
If sustained, these can all impair CO significantly and even lead to cardiac arrest. The same applies to massive pulmonary embolism impairing VR to the left heart. Mitral stenosis has a similar effect.

A4 • A decrease in inotropy (force of contraction) as seen in cardiac failure, leads to a fall in stroke volume and an increase in preload. This is demonstrated by a shift to the right in the Starling curve. If the increased preload results in a left ventricular end-diastolic pressure greater than 20 mmHg, it can lead to pulmonary oedema.
  • Compensatory mechanisms take effect in cardiac failure. Activation of sympathetic nerves and the rennin–angiotensin system, and increased release of antidiuretic hormone (vasopressin) and atrial natriuretic peptide produce arterial vasoconstriction (to help maintain arterial pressure), venous constriction (increased venous pressure), and increased blood volume.

- These mechanisms can also aggravate heart failure by increasing ventricular afterload (which depresses stroke volume) and increasing preload to the point where pulmonary or systemic congestion and oedema occur. When afterload increases, there is an increase in end-systolic volume and a decrease in stroke volume. An increase in afterload *per se* shifts the Frank–Starling curve down and to the right, as occurs in cardiac failure.

- Treating a patient in heart failure with an inotropic drug will shift the Starling curve up and to the left, thereby increasing stroke volume, decreasing preload, and increasing CO. A variety of inotropic drugs are used clinically to stimulate the heart, particularly in acute and chronic heart failure. These drugs include digoxin, which inhibits sarcolemmal N^+/K^+-ATPase, beta-adrenoceptor agonists, e.g. adrenaline, dopamine, dobutamine and phosphodiesterase inhibitors, e.g. milrinone. Other treatment modalities in cardiac failure include diuretics, vasodilators and beta-blockers. The sympathetic nervous system is activated in patients with heart failure, and the judicious use of beta-blockers, which inhibit sympathetic activity, might reduce the risk of disease progression.

Your revision notes:

Abdominal compartment syndrome (ACS)

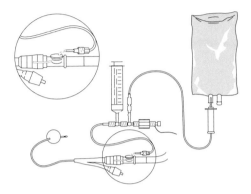

Figure 2.13

Questions

Q1 How is ACS diagnosed?

Q2 What is the cause of raised intra-abdominal pressure?

Q3 Under what circumstances should the diagnosis of ACS be entertained?

Q4 What are the possible means of diagnosing ACS?

Q5 What are the effects of ACS on various organ systems?

Q6 What levels of pressure cause concern?

Q7 What is the treatment? What is the risk of treatment?

Answers

(A1) Intra-abdominal hypertension (IAH) is most often monitored with intravesical pressure measurement (as above) to diagnose ACS.

(A2) The ACS represents the pathophysiological consequence of moderate to severe raised intra-abdominal pressure. The multiple trauma patient, with massive intra-abdominal or retroperitoneal haemorrhage and placement of intra-abdominal packs to control bleeding is a common cause. Severe intestinal oedema of whatever cause, or intestinal obstruction, and ascites under pressure are other well-known causes. Ruptured AAA patients, who have had prolonged surgery and large volume resuscitation, should also be kept in mind.

(A3) When confronted with a patient with circulatory failure and elevated filling pressures – CVP or PCWP – it is imperative to exclude pericardial tamponade and increased pleural pressure (tension pneumothorax, status asthmaticus, etc). However the ACS should be kept in mind and excluded by pressure measurement.

(A4) • A high index of suspicion should be kept in mind in the clinical scenarios mentioned above. However physical signs are misleading.
• Measurement of intravesical, inferior vena cava, rectal and gastric pressure reflects indirectly on IAP. Direct measurement of the IAP by direct puncture is sometimes possible but fraught with many problems and complications. In experimental conditions, bladder pressure is closely related to abdominal pressure and has become the most commonly used modality in clinical practice.

(A5) **Cardiovascular system**
IAH has been shown to decrease cardiac output despite elevated CVP. Reduction in venous return to the heart appears a major problem. Volume challenge improves these parameters slightly, but only abdominal decompression results in significant improvement in cardiac function. Laparotomy with decompression markedly reduces CVP and PCWP and increases cardiac output.

Pulmonary and respiratory systems
Elevated peak inspiratory pressures, decreases in PaO_2 and increases in $PaCO_2$ are often seen early on. The rises in peak airway pressure and intrathoracic pressure cause reduced venous return to the heart. The increase in airway pressures may also exacerbate pulmonary barotrauma. Peak airway pressure improves to near normal levels immediately after surgical decompression of the abdomen.

Renal system
Renal effects of IAH and ACS include decreased renal plasma flow and glomerular filtration rate, and oliguria or anuria. Improvement in renal function occurs only after abdominal decompression. It is suggested that the effects of IAH on renal function are related to compression of the renal parenchyma itself and to compression of renal vasculature, and are not only related to decreased cardiac output.

(A6) IAP is normally 0 mmHg to subatmospheric, but may increase to 15 mmHg after abdominal surgery. IAH is defined as IAP higher than 15–20 mmHg (20–25 cmH_2O if a water manometer is used).

(A7) • A laparotomy is done for decompression of established ACS. However patients are at risk of developing sudden, severe hypotension immediately after the abdominal cavity is opened. A sudden decrease in effective preload from re-expansion of abdominal and pelvic veins and from washout of anaerobic products is postulated.
• Anticipating the development of ACS and the use of an alternative wound closure technique, could prevent its occurrence.

Porphyria

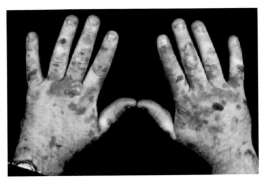

Figure 2.14

Questions

Q1 A patient with acute abdominal pain is noticed to also have a bullous rash on the hands. What is the diagnosis?

Q2 What is porphyria?

Q3 How does porphyria present?

Q4 How do you diagnose porphyria?

Q5 What is the management of an acute porphyria attack?

Answers

 An acute attack of porphyria should be kept in mind in patients with abdominal pain with a bullous rash, or scarring of the sun-exposed areas of the body.

- The porphyrias are disorders of the haem biosynthetic pathway. They present with acute abdominal or neurological crises or skin lesions or a combination of these. All porphyrias result from partial deficiency of one of the enzymes of haem biosynthesis. Acute porphyria occurs in three similar presentations: acute intermittent porphyria (AIP), variegate porphyria (VP) and hereditary coproporphyria (HCP). They are grouped together because acute attacks of porphyria occur in each one. They are inherited in autosomal dominant fashion, and asymptomatic gene carriers are often encountered.
- In most European countries, about 1 in 75 000 people suffer from porphyria. In Northern Scandinavia and certain parts of South Africa it is much more common. Acute intermittent porphyria is the commonest type. In this disease, only acute attacks occur and the skin is spared leaving no warning stigmata for the alert clinician. In VP or HCP, the skin may also be affected.

 Attacks are often provoked by drugs, alcohol, starvation, endocrine factors or infection. The most common triggering drugs are barbiturates, sulphonamides and anticonvulsants. Acute abdominal pain, vomiting and constipation may imitate an acute abdominal condition. This may be associated with autonomic disturbances like hypertension and tachycardia. Various neuropsychological symptoms may further confuse the issue. Porphyria should always be considered if acute abdominal pain occurs in a patient labelled as hysterical. Keep this diagnosis in mind in cases where a negative laparotomy was found. Hyponatraemia, convulsions and airway problems could contribute to a fatal outcome.

- Acute attacks are accompanied by increased urinary excretion of porphobilinogen (PBG) and, to a lesser extent, amino-laevulinic acid (ALA). If urinary PBG and ALA, plasma porphyrin concentration and faecal coproporphyrin III excretion are normal, acute porphyria is excluded as the cause of acute symptoms. Urinary PBG is best analysed in a fresh, random sample (10–20 ml) collected without any preservative, but protected from light.
- Most patients with an attack of acute porphyria have PBG concentrations at least ten times the upper limit of normal within one week of the onset of symptoms. At these concentrations, urine samples may develop a brownish red colour (port-wine) on standing. During remission, the diagnosis may be difficult because urinary, faecal and plasma porphyrin concentrations may return to normal. Furthermore neither enzyme measurements nor mutational analysis is 100% sensitive and 100% specific.
- In all patients, urinary PBG and ALA excretion should be determined, if negative then faecal porphyrins should be analysed. Plasma porphyrin fluorescence emission spectrum and erythrocyte PBG deaminase activity may also be helpful.

- *Supportive treatment* using safe drugs is the cornerstone of treatment. Withdraw any causative drugs or other potential causative agents. Attention to fluid balance is essential. Avoid large volumes of hypotonic dextrose, to prevent the risk of hyponatraemia which may provoke convulsions. Hyponatraemia should be corrected slowly if it occurs. Patients with acute attacks seem particularly prone to cerebral oedema and osmotic demyelination.

- Adequate calories should be given early, since impaired nutrition may aggravate acute porphyria. Carbohydrate-rich food supplements should preferably be given orally or via a nasogastric tube. When vomiting prevents enteral administration, carbohydrate may be provided intravenously.
- Muscle weakness progressing to paralysis may necessitate artificial ventilation. It may have to be continued for several months until the expected eventual recovery occurs.
- *Specific treatment* should be started as soon as the diagnosis is established unless the attack is mild and clearly resolving. Two treatments are available: intravenous haem arginate and carbohydrate loading. Intravenous haem is the more effective and should be used unless it is not available. Neither will reverse an established peripheral neuropathy, though haem may prevent its onset and may halt further progression of neuropathy if given sufficiently early.

Your revision notes:

Enteral nutrition

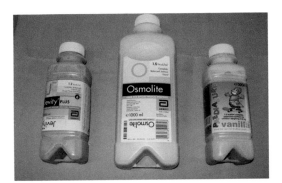

Figure 2.15

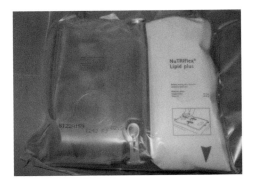

Figure 2.16

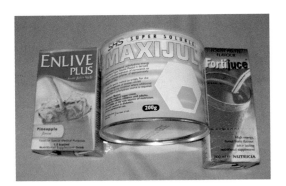

Figure 2.17

Figure 2.15 shows examples of enteral nutrition, Figure 2.16 examples of parenteral nutrition and Figure 2.17 examples of nutritional supplements. The following questions relate to enteral nutrition in the surgical patient.

Questions

Q1 What are the advantages of enteral nutrition?

Q2 What are the different ways to maintain enteral nutrition?

Q3 What are some of the conditions where enteral feeding may not be possible (what are the indications for parenteral feeding)?

Q4 What are the different types of diets that are given by the enteral route?

Q5 What are some of the complications associated with enteral feeding?

Answers

 • Prevents mucosal atrophy.
- Reduces bacterial translocation from the gut, which has been considered as a cause for respiratory and other infections.
- Reduces the release of cytokines from unused gut.
- More physiological compared to parenteral nutrition.
- Avoids all complications of central line placement.

 • Normal oral intake.
- Fine-bore nasogastric feeding tube.
- Nasojejunal tube.
- Percutaneous endoscopic gastrostomy tube.
- Percutaneous endoscopic jejunostomy tube.
- Intra-operative placement of feeding gastrostomy/jejunostomy tube.

 • Intestinal obstruction.
- Non-availability of intestine as in short gut syndrome.
- In cases of enterocutaneous fistula.
- In the immediate post-operative period, in the presence of ileus.
- Where it is not possible to provide sufficient calories via the enteral route, the parenteral route may be additionally needed, as in severe trauma or in burns.

 Enteral feeds are broadly divided into three categories:
- *polymeric diets*: these contain whole protein as a nitrogen source, triglycerides and glucose polymers as an energy source, and standardised amounts of electrolytes, trace elements and vitamins. This type of diet is usually prescribed in patients with normal or near-normal GI function
- *predigested or elemental diet*: these contain free amino acids or oligopeptides as a nitrogen source, short-chain (>10) glucose polymers as an energy source and long- and medium-chain triglycerides as a fat source. These diets are preferred in patients with severe pancreatitis, or in short bowel syndrome
- *disease-specific diets*: these are specially formulated diets avoiding ingredients that can worsen an encephalopathy or respiratory failure.

 • Even though enteral feeding has many advantages, complications can result from feeding tube placement or directly related to the diet itself. Complications related to tube placement include malposition of the tube, unwanted removal and blockage of the tube.
- Diet-related complications include drug interactions, abdominal bloating, diarrhoea, cramps, regurgitation and pulmonary aspiration, and vitamin, mineral and trace element deficiencies.

Fat embolism syndrome

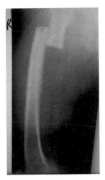

Figure 2.18

A 50-year-old gentleman was involved in a road traffic accident. Twenty-four hours following admission he developed sudden onset shortness of breath, pyrexia and a tachycardia.

Questions

Q1 Describe what the plain film shows.

Q2 What is the clinical diagnosis?

Q3 What are the other clinical features to look for?

Q4 What are the other predisposing factors for developing this problem?

Q5 What is the treatment?

Answers

A1 There is a transverse fracture through the proximal third of the right femur (diaphysis), with gross displacement, angulation and overlap of the fracture fragments.

A2 Fat embolism (from bone marrow). This occurs in 90% of patients who sustain significant skeletal trauma.

A3
- *Symptoms*: mental confusion due to cerebral oedema and microinfarcts. May start with just irritability and restlessness.
- *Signs*: tachycardia, unexplained pyrexia (usually 12–24 h after injury; too early to be infective), hypercapnia and hypoxia, raised RR, petechiae on the front and back of the chest and in the conjunctival folds (20–50%).
- *Severe cases*: respiratory distress and coma.
- Thrombocytopaenia and anaemia may occur.

A4 Burns, soft tissue trauma, renal infarction, hyperlipidaemia, pancreatitis, ischaemic marrow necrosis in sickle cell disease and cardiopulmonary operations.

A5
- Mild cases: no treatment is required but serial examination and close monitoring are required, with arterial blood gases and fluid balance.
- Severe respiratory distress will require intensive care support.
- PEEP can re-open collapsed alveoli.
- Neither heparin or steroids have any proven benefit.
- 10% of cases are fatal.

Section 3

Transplant and

vascular access

Radiocephalic AV fistula

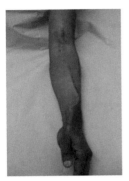

Figure 3.1

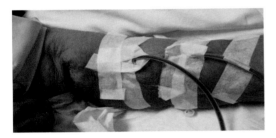

Figure 3.2

Questions

Q1 What is the spot diagnosis and what is it used for? (Figure 3.1)

Q2 Describe the clinical signs.

Q3 What are the favoured sites for the formation of an AV fistula?

Q4 Describe the AV fistula site shown in Figure 3.2 and other options available for access.

Answers

 Radiocephalic AV fistula used as vascular access for haemodialysis.

 • *Inspection*: visible enlarged cephalic vein. If there is evidence of puncture marks from needling then this will confirm that this has been used for haemodialysis.
• *Palpation*: characteristic thrill or buzz 'like a mobile phone on vibrate mode'.
• *Percussion*: transmissible tap test.
• *Auscultation*: machinery murmur or continuous bruit.

 Snuff box: radial artery to cephalic vein.
• The forearm: radial artery to cephalic vein, also known as a Brescia–Cimino fistula.
• The antecubital fossa: brachial artery to cephalic vein, also known as a brachio-cephalic fistula.
• The non-dominant hand is chosen preferentially, to free the dominant hand for use during haemodialysis sessions. The first fistula formed tends to be as distal as possible to preserve the vessels further up the arm for future access.

 • Brachiobasilic fistula between the brachial artery and the basilic vein. The upper arm basilic vein runs a deep course under the fascia above the antecubital fossa. This would therefore make it awkward to needle and position the needles for the haemodialysis sessions. It is therefore necessary to superficialise and transpose the basilic vein so that it lies in an accessible position in the forearm.
• Other possible sites/options include an autogenous vein and an artificial graft.
• An autogenous vein is preferred as there is a reduced risk of infection.
• If the cephalic vein is <2 mm then this is unlikely to mature to form a suitable fistula and it is appropriate to look at other veins. The basilic vein, which runs a superficial course in the medial side of the forearm, can be used:
  – the forearm ulnobasilic vein between the ulnar artery and the basilic vein
  – the forearm radiobasilic vein between the radial artery and the basilic vein. This will need mobilisation and transposition of the forearm basilic vein
  – the brachiobasilic vein as demonstrated can be used as an option.
• If the veins in the arms have been exhausted, then the next option is to look at the legs. The saphenous vein in the legs can be used either as an *in situ* graft from the popliteal artery, anastomosing the popliteal artery to the saphenous vein, or as a leg loop graft between the mobilised saphenous vein which has formed a loop to the femoral artery.
• If there are no suitable veins for access then the next option is to use an artificial graft such as PTFE or Dacron. There are some newer grafts which have been used for access. The sites can be anywhere that is superficial where an artery and a vein can be joined up with a graft.

Vascular catheters

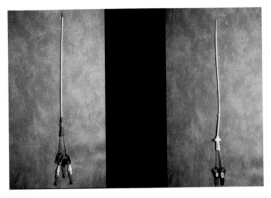

Figure 3.3

Questions

Q1 What are these two instruments used for?

Q2 What are the differences between the two catheters?

Q3 Which vessels should be used for cannulation?

Q4 What are the potential complications of insertion of these lines?

Q5 What are the complications of an indwelling TDC?

Answers

 Vascular access catheters for haemodialysis.

 • One catheter has three lumens with no cuff and is used as a temporary means of providing haemodialysis (no more than 5–7 days).
• The second catheter is a tunnelled dialysis catheter (TDC) which has two ports and a cuff which serves two purposes. One is to secure the line by stimulating a fibrous response in the adjacent tissue of the subcutaneous tunnel, which then anchors itself to the catheter. The second purpose is to prevent migration of skin commensals and other bacteria to cause infection. For this reason the TDC can be used for dialysis for longer periods.

 • The right internal jugular vein is the vessel of choice since this has a direct route to the SVC and right atrium.
• If the left internal jugular is used then this will involve passing the cannula around the innominate vein, and the tip of both ports should be positioned in the SVC.
• The external jugulars can be used for insertion of a TDC, but final positioning of the tips needs to be in the SVC.
• The left and right femoral veins are then chosen.
• The subclavian veins should be avoided as there is an increased risk of stenosis, and this will compromise the ipsilateral arm for a more definitive access procedure.

 • Haemorrhage.
• Pneumothorax.
• Haemothorax.
• Air embolus.
• Cardiac arrhythmias.
• Inadvertent cannulation of the carotid artery.
• Traumatic AV fistula.
• Nerve injury.
• Malposition of the line.
• Malfunction of the line.

 • *Thrombosis*: each port needs to be primed with heparin at the end of dialysis to prevent this complication. If this fails then sometimes a thrombolytic agent such as tPA is used. It is essential to aspirate this before commencing dialysis, otherwise the patient will inadvertently be given a bolus which may render them coagulopathic.
• *Embolisation*: thrombi may form on the end of the catheter and propagate. This could cause a pulmonary embolus. If the ports are not primed or left open then they may develop an air embolus.
• *Mechanical*: if the TDC migrates or becomes kinked then it will no longer function. Sometimes the tip of one of the ports abuts against the side wall of the vessel and it simply needs to be pulled back.
• *Infection*: the catheter itself could become infected locally with tunnel site infections or infections of the catheter itself. This could rapidly progress to distant complications such as endocarditis, septic emboli and septicaemia. The management of this is to remove the catheter as soon as possible and treat with antibiotics. A new temporary line should be inserted into a different site after a few days of remaining free from prosthetic material.
• *Venous stenosis*: if left indwelling for prolonged periods there is also a risk of stenosis to the vein. This may progress to SVC occlusion but the main problem is the development of venous hypertension in the ipsilateral limb and compromised vascular access options in that limb.

PD catheters

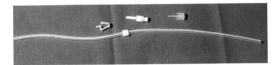

Figure 3.4

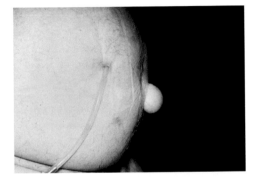

Figure 3.5

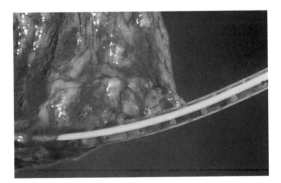

Figure 3.6

Questions

Q1 What is the tube in Figure 3.4 called and what is it used for?

Q2 Describe the features of the tube.

Q3 How is renal replacement therapy carried out using this tube?

Q4 What complications are demonstrated using this form of dialysis (Figures 3.5 and 3.6)? What other complications can occur?

Q5 What are the relative benefits and disadvantages of this modality of dialysis compared to haemodialysis?

Answers

 A Tenckhoff catheter, and it is used for peritoneal dialysis.

 A hollow tube made from inert material (silastic) which at one end has multiple holes for draining fluid easily. There are two cuffs made of Dacron which form part of the tube to anchor the tube in position (at the pre-peritoneal site of entry into the peritoneum and a few centimetres from the skin exit site). These cuffs also prevent migration of skin commensals and other bacteria along the catheter.

 • The fluid and solute transport characteristics of the peritoneum, which serves as an endogenous dialysis membrane, are used.
• Access to the peritoneal cavity is achieved using this catheter, and the tip of the catheter is placed in the pelvis.
• A specified volume of dialysing fluid is instilled into the peritoneal cavity by gravity-induced flow. The fluid is then allowed to dwell for a period during which solute removal and ultrafiltration are achieved. The fluid is then drained and discarded. The process is then repeated.
• In continuous ambulatory peritoneal dialysis (CAPD) the patient exchanges the bags themselves and the dialysis continues 24 h per day with four to five exchanges per day. In continuous cycling peritoneal dialysis (CCPD) or automated peritoneal dialysis (APD), an automated cycling device is used to regulate and monitor the dialysate flow into and out of the abdomen, and four to ten exchanges are performed nightly over 8–10 h.

 Umbilical hernia formation (Figure 3.5): the increased intra-abdominal pressure may predispose to the formation of herniae, subcutaneous leaks or even pleural effusions if there are congenital diaphragmatic herniae.
• Figure 3.6 demonstrates *occlusion of the tube by omentum*. This will result in failure of instillation of PD fluid or drainage of the fluid from the peritoneum.
• For this reason some centres practise omentectomy at the time of PD catheter insertion.
• *Other mechanical problems* can occur, resulting in failure of instillation or drainage of fluid. This could be due to kinking of the tube, external compression, for example by a constipated sigmoid colon and rectum, or the tip of the PD catheter may have flipped out from the pelvis making it more difficult to drain fluid.
• *Infection* of exit site, tunnel or peritoneum.
• *Malfunction* of dialysis: due to peritoneal membrane failure, lack of an adequate peritoneal membrane or due to the presence of numerous adhesions minimising the space in the peritoneum for fluid.

 • Maintenance of relatively constant blood or serum levels of urea, creatinine and electrolytes using PD.
• Better blood pressure control with PD.
• Dialysate is a form of nutrition.
• Promotes self-care and independence.
• Can allow a more liberal diet with PD compared to strict diet and treatment schedules.
• Haemodialysis allows a comparatively shorter treatment time.
• Haemodialysis allows ongoing social interaction for patients with little support.

Sclerosing peritonitis

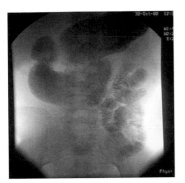

Figure 3.7

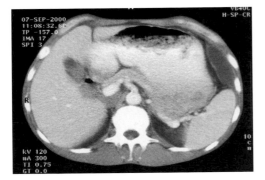

Figure 3.8

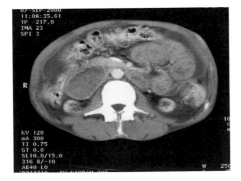

Figure 3.9

This is a study of a 38-year-old male who has had three years of PD.

Questions

Q1 What is this investigation (Figure 3.7) and what abnormalities does it show?

Q2 Which clinical features might this cause?

Q3 The CT scans in Figures 3.8 and 3.9 were performed in the same patient. What are the radiological abnormalities?

Q4 What is the differential diagnosis?

Q5 What is the management?

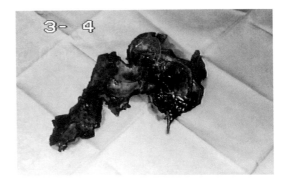

Figure 3.10

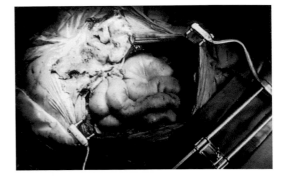

Figure 3.11

Answers

(A1) This is a barium meal with follow-through which demonstrates a grossly distended stomach and duodenum.

(A2)
- *Symptoms*: vomiting undigested food products and bile, weight loss and failure to thrive, abdominal pain and distension.
- *Signs*: malnourished, dehydrated, tachycardia, abdominal distension, succussion splash.

(A3) Cystic abnormality in the abdomen, thickened peritoneum and thickened small bowel.

(A4)
- Abscess.
- Peritoneal cyst.
- Mesenteric cyst.
- Pseudomyxoma peritonei.
- Peritoneal fluid collection which has become encysted.
- Sclerosing peritonitis.

(A5) For sclerosing peritonitis the management is divided into conservative treatment, medical treatment with the use of azathioprine and tamoxifen, and surgical treatment. Laparotomy should be delayed until a period of hyperalimentation. The laparotomy findings often find a thickened peritoneum with chronic changes to the small bowel giving it a tanned, leathery appearance. There may also be encasement by a fibrous cocoon or rusk which can cause a more aggressive form of this condition known as sclerosing encapsulating peritonitis (see laparotomy findings in a different patient – Figures 3.10 and 3.11).
The cocoon is carefully removed from the serosa of the small bowel and any other fibrous tissue causing obstruction should also be excised.

Complications of AV fistulae

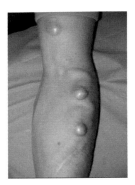

Figure 3.12

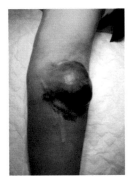

Figure 3.14

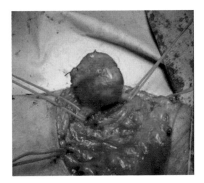

Figure 3.13

Questions

Q1 What is the diagnosis for Figure 3.12 and what has caused this?

Q2 What are the complications shown in Figures 3.13 and 3.14, and how can these be distinguished clinically?

Q3 How should the conditions shown in Figures 3.13 and 3.14 be managed?

Q4 What are the other specific complications of AV fistula formation?

Answers

(A1) Aneurysms of the arterialised vein. These have been caused by repetitive puncturing of the vein in the same site, known as 'buttonholing'. This technique should be avoided in artificial grafts as there would be a significant risk of rupture. Instead the site of needling should be staggered ('laddering').

(A2)
- In the aneurysm (Figure 3.13), the dilated part contains all three walls of the blood vessel (intima, media and adventitia), and the dilated portion has an expansile pulse.
- In the pseudoaneurysm (Figure 3.14), the wall of the dilated part contains clot and not the three layers of the blood vessel.

(A3)
- *Aneurysm* (Figure 3.13): if expanding significantly or causing other symptoms then the aneurysm should be resected. This could be performed either with ligation of the fistula or by attempting to preserve the fistula so that it could be used for subsequent access.
- *Pseudoaneurysm* (Figure 3.14): in the acute situation direct pressure over the leak with the main vessel may be of benefit. Sometimes an ultrasound probe may be used for direct pressure, with the added benefit of accurate visualisation of the abnormal communication. If this fails to control the aneurysm then radiological stenting may be of use or even open surgery to close the defect.

(A4)
- Failure to mature.
- Stenosis.
- Thrombosis.
- Venous hypertension.
- Steal phenomenon.
- High-output cardiac failure.
- Ischaemic monomelic neuropathy.

Renal transplant incision

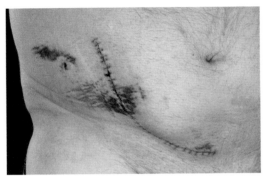

Figure 3.15

Questions

Q1 What is this incision and what is this used for?

Q2 What is the differential diagnosis of a mass in the right iliac fossa?

Q3 Is this a heterotopic transplant or an othotopic transplant, and what are the differences?

Q4 During this operation which anastomoses are performed?

Q5 From what donor source do these kidneys come?

Answers

 A hockey stick incision for renal transplantation.

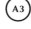
- Kidney transplant – with accompanying incision.
- Ovarian tumour.
- Caecal tumour.
- Appendix mass.
- Iliac aneurysm.
- Inguinal hernia.
- Lipoma.
- Sebaceous cyst.
- Neurofibroma.
- Rhabdomyofibroma.

 This is a heterotopic transplant as the new kidney is put into a different position to where the native kidneys are, and these are not removed.

- Renal artery to external iliac artery or internal iliac artery.
- Renal vein to external iliac vein.
- Ureter to bladder.

- *A living donor* who can be related or unrelated to the recipient.
- *A cadaveric or deceased donor:* these donors can be divided into brainstem death donors who will become heart-beating donors, and donors who do not fulfil the brainstem death criteria.

Renal transplant complicated by lymphocoele

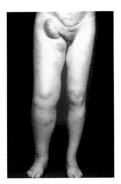

Figure 3.16

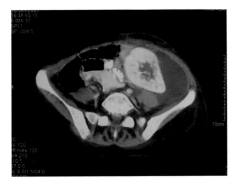

Figure 3.18

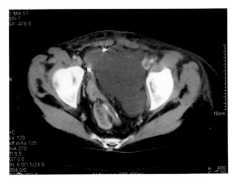

Figure 3.17

Questions

Q1 What two clinical signs are seen in this patient (Figure 3.16) who has had a recent renal transplant?

Q2 What is the differential diagnosis for these two clinical findings?

Q3 How should a definitive diagnosis be made?

Q4 Describe the radiological abnormalities (Figures 3.17 and 3.18) in this separate patient who had a transplant four weeks earlier.

Answers

 A1 There are two main clinical findings on inspection. These are the presence of a discoloured right groin swelling and the unilateral right leg swelling.

 A2 **Groin swelling**
- Inguinal hernia.
- Femoral hernia.
- Haematoma.
- Lymphocoele / seroma.
- Enlarged LN.
- Saphena varix.
- Abscess.
- Femoral artery aneurysm/pseudoaneurysm.
- Urinoma.

Unilateral leg swelling
- Deep venous thrombosis.
- Lymphoedema.
- Venous congestion caused by extrinsic pressure on the iliac femoral vein.
- Post-thrombotic leg swelling.

 A3 The diagnosis should be obvious after a thorough history, clinical examination and investigations of the groin swelling and leg swelling.

History
- Did the groin swelling precede the transplant?
- Did the leg swelling precede the transplant?
- Is there any previous history of deep venous thrombosis?
- If the groin swelling was present before the transplant, was it reducible? Did it have a cough impulse?
- Any other symptoms suggestive of pelvic compression such as urinary frequency or constipation?

Examination
- *Groin*:
  - inspection: cough impulse?
  - palpation: tender? warm? reducible? cough impulse? transmitted pulse? expansile pulse?
  - percussion
  - auscultation: bruit? bowel sounds?
- *Leg*:
  - inspection: chronic changes of venous hypertension?
  - palpation: warm? tender? pitting or non-pitting oedema?

Investigations
- An ultrasound of the groin swelling will be able to identify if the groin swelling contains fluid, and also the leg veins can be imaged to rule out a deep venous thrombosis. If a collection is present then this can be aspirated for biochemistry and microbiology. If there is doubt as to whether it is urine or lymph/serum, the creatinine level would give a fair indication of this. The urinary creatinine is >5 mmol/l whereas the level in

lymphatic fluid is similar to that of serum (micromol/l). Furthermore, the glucose content in the serum/lymph would be the same as in serum, whereas it should be negative in urine (except in diabetics). Finally the protein content in lymph/serum should be >20 g/l compared to urine which should be <1 g/l.

- In this particular patient this was a cystic collection which contained lymph. The diagnosis was therefore a lymphocoele. There was venous compression in this patient but fortunately there was no deep venous thrombosis.

 CT scan at two levels.

- At the level of the iliac crest there is a collection lateral to the transplant kidney. In the CT scan at the level of the femoral heads there are more abnormalities. There is a spherical circular collection which has caused compression and deviation of the bladder. Inside the bladder the urinary stent is seen. This central structure is also causing compression of the rectum. The iliac vein is also seen with evidence of thrombus within the lumen. In summary this collection has caused bladder and bowel compression and is likely to have contributed to venous stasis and caused a deep venous thrombosis. The presence of the ureteric stent has probably prevented ureteric obstruction of the transplant kidney.
- The collection in the image lateral to the kidney was demonstrated to be communicating with the deep pelvic collection (not shown) and the diagnosis was subsequently confirmed to be a lymphocoele.

Your revision notes:

Renal transplant complicated by renal vein thrombosis

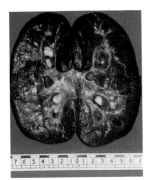

Figure 3.19

Questions

Q1 What has occurred in this graft nephrectomy?

Q2 What factors predispose to this?

Q3 How may the condition present?

Q4 What is the management?

Q5 What is the differential diagnosis that could be prevented by a cross-match, and how is this performed?

Answers

A1 The specimen demonstrates a swollen congested graft nephrectomy with evidence of thrombus in the renal vein. This represents a renal vein thrombosis.

A2 This can be summarised by Virchow's triad:
1 *alteration in blood flow*: during a renal transplant there is stagnation of flow across the iliac vein when the vessels are clamped for the renal vein anastomosis. In the post-operative period, alterations in the blood pressure such as hypotension will cause reduced perfusion of the kidney
2 *alteration in the constituents of blood*: it is often observed that renal failure patients have a co-existing thrombophilia as evidenced by the coagulation of vascular access grafts. This could be due to a primary cause of hypercoagulability (such as protein C, protein S or antithrombin III deficiency or factor V Leiden mutation) or more commonly a secondary cause of hypercoagulability (such as antiphospholipid syndrome)
3 *damage to the vessel wall*: this is relevant during a renal transplant where the renal vessels could be damaged during the retrieval process, the benchwork preparation of the kidney or during the implantation. Care has to be taken to avoid trauma to the renal vein, with careful application of the vessel clamps to the iliac vein, minimal instrumentation of the intima during the anastomosis, and careful positioning of the venous sutures to avoid any stenoses or kinks that might be thrombogenic.

A3 The condition presents with a sudden decrease in the renal output in the early post-operative period. This may be accompanied with haematuria and pain over the renal graft. A duplex ultrasound would demonstrate renal vein thrombosis with reverse flow during diastole. If the condition progresses this could even lead to rupture of the kidney with a catastrophic loss of blood from the kidney.

A4 The condition occurs in approximately 1% of kidney transplants. The early diagnosis of a sudden loss of urine output with a duplex ultrasound may allow a surgical thrombectomy. Unfortunately at surgery there is little that can be done and this is managed with a graft nephrectomy. There is some evidence to suggest thrombolysis may have a role, but the risks of catastrophic bleeding from a recently formed anastomosis outweigh the potential benefits.

A5 Hyperacute rejection: this is a rare and largely preventable cause of immediate graft failure. It is caused by the presence of preformed antibodies in the recipient serum to donor antigens which would have developed by previous exposure to those antigens by blood transfusions, previous transplantation or pregnancy. This type of reaction can also occur if an ABO-incompatible transplant is inadvertently performed.
- There are two types of cross-match test:
  - *complement-dependent cytotoxicity* (CDC): lymphocytes (T and B) from the donor are incubated with serum from the recipient at room temperature, 37°C, and in the cold at 4°C. Rabbit complement is added to cause cell lysis. After 3 h of incubation the cells are inspected for evidence of killing. If the recipient's serum (in the presence of rabbit complement) kills the donor lymphocytes, then a preformed antibody is present and the cross-match is recorded as positive. This means the transplant is contraindicated
  - *flow cytometry*: donor lymphocytes are incubated first with recipient serum and then with a fluorescent-labelled polyvalent anti-IgG antibody. If the recipient antibody to donor lymphocytes is present, it will be detected by the flow cytometer. This cross-match test is more sensitive than the CDC test.

Renal artery stenosis

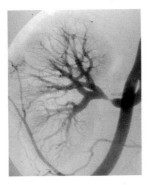

Figure 3.20

Questions

Q1 What is this investigation and how is it carried out?

Q2 What are the radiological findings?

Q3 How might this patient present?

Q4 Describe the non-invasive means of diagnosis.

Q5 How should this be managed?

Answers

A1 Digital subtraction angiogram of a renal transplant: the ipsilateral or contralateral femoral artery is cannulated and a guidewire is inserted and manoeuvred into position. This is then exchanged for a further cannula, and radiopaque contrast is injected into the vessel.

A2 This demonstrates that the renal artery is anastomosed to the internal iliac artery, but at the region of the anastomosis there is a stenosis.

A3 The condition should be suspected in renal transplants where there was a difficult anastomosis with small, diseased or multiple donor vessels. The patient is likely to present with increasingly difficult to manage hypertension with the use of more antihypertensive agents. There may also be a deterioration in the renal function, with an elevated creatinine possibly precipitated by an ACE inhibitor. Occasionally there may be episodes of flash pulmonary oedema. On clinical examination there may be a new transplant bruit.

A4 The clinical finding of uncontrolled hypertension on numerous antihypertensives with a new transplant bruit is highly suggestive of the diagnosis. Non-invasive investigations include a duplex ultrasound, MRA and a pre- and post-captopril renogram.

A5 Transplant renal artery stenosis is diagnosed in approximately 2% of renal transplant recipients. The definitive diagnosis is made on intra-arterial DSA. Percutaneous transluminal angioplasty is the usual initial intervention and is successful in up to 85% of the procedures, but there is often a re-stenosis rate. If this fails then surgical reperfusion by re-implanting onto the internal iliac artery or a jump graft using the saphenous vein can be performed, but this is complex surgery due to the dense scar tissue around the transplant, and there is a risk of graft loss.

Laparoscopic organ donation

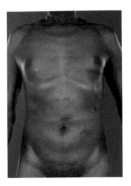

Figure 3.21

Questions

Q1 What procdure has been carried out in this patient?

Q2 What investigations should be carried out in this patient before deciding it is safe to proceed to surgery?

Q3 Which factors influence the side of surgery?

Q4 What are the benefits to the donor from this type of surgery?

Answers

 Laparoscopic donor nephrectomy.

 The donor has an extensive work-up prior to confirming suitability for donor nephrectomy and in practice this is divided into several phases:

- *phase 1*: initial assessment with blood group testing to ensure ABO compatibility, HLA tissue typing and cross-match to ensure immunological compatibility
- *phase 2*: history, examination and investigations of the potential donor including a comprehensive range of blood tests (haematology, biochemistry and virology) and urine tests (biochemistry and microbiology). The potential donor then undergoes a series of scans including an ultrasound (to confirm two kidneys), nuclear medicine GFR (to assess overall renal function), DMSA to check relative contribution to total function by each kidney
- *phase 3*: review of the above investigations and if OK an arteriogram is performed as a roadmap for the vasculature to both kidneys. This could be as an invasive DSA with selective cannulation of each renal artery to rule out anomalous vessels, or non-invasive, as a CT or MRI scan with three-dimensional reconstructions. A final cross-match between the donor and recipient is usually performed within a few weeks of surgery.

- This can be influenced by donor factors, surgeon's preference and to a lesser extent recipient factors which would become apparent during the work-up process. However the basic principle is to accommodate the donor's wishes but also to prevent them from being potentially compromised in the future.
- The arteriogram determines the number of arteries to each kidney. Anomalous anatomy may make both donor nephrectomy and the recipient transplant more complicated.
- The DMSA scan may indicate a discrepant renal function between the kidneys, and if this is the case then the kidney with poorer function should be removed.
- If both kidneys have a single artery and vein with similar function, then the left side is preferentially removed on the grounds that it has a longer renal vein making the recipient procedure more straightforward.
- An ultrasound may demonstrate a benign abnormality in the kidney such as a simple cyst, which may influence the surgeon or the donor on the choice of side.
- Recipient factors that may influence the choice of graft nephrectomy in the donor could be the sex of the recipient (males have a narrow pelvis with deeper vessels), the weight of the recipient (if overweight then the surgeon will prefer longer vessels), and the proposed transplantation site (the iliac vessels tend to lie more deeply on the left side than the right).

- There are numerous benefits to the donor which include reduced pain from the procedure, with fewer opiates required for a shorter duration, reduced hospital admission and earlier return to activities of daily living as well as work. The incidence of chest-related and wound-related complications is also thought to be reduced.
- There has been discussion of potential complications, but these have yet to be validated in a randomised controlled study. The potential complications are thought to be due to a prolonged ischaemic time between clamping the renal artery and flushing out the blood from the kidney with preservation fluid, which may lead to a delay in the kidney starting to work (delayed graft function). It has been postulated also that the laparoscopic process may potentially damage the renal vessels and the ureter.
- Although there is no doubt that there is a learning curve associated with the procedure, this should be regarded as a safe procedure in the hands of an experienced laparoscopic team.

Liver transplant incision

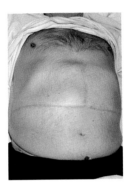

Figure 3.22

Questions

Q1 What is this incision and what is it used for?

Q2 What are the indications for this procedure?

Q3 What are the steps of this procedure, and which anastomoses are performed?

Q4 What are the potential complications of this procedure?

Answers

 This is a Mercedes–Benz incision which is used for a liver transplant. Other incisions can be used for this procedure including an 'inverted T', a 'reverse L', a 'rooftop' or 'subcostal' incision.

 These can be classified broadly into four categories:
1 chronic liver disease with end-stage liver failure
2 acute liver failure
3 liver malignancy where a conventional resection is not possible
4 to replace a defective liver enzyme.

 This is an orthotopic transplant where the liver is removed and the donor liver is implanted into the same site. The procedure can be divided into the following stages:
- *donor hepatectomy*: this is performed in advance of the recipient procedure and usually a retrieval team is sent to the donor hospital to retrieve the liver. This is often as part of multiple-organ retrieval, and there may be a kidney team, a pancreatic team and a cardiothoracic team. The liver is retrieved, flushed with cold preservation fluid and kept cool by storing 'on ice'. It is then transported to the recipient hospital
- *backbench preparation of the donor liver*: the liver is inspected for quality and to prepare it for implantation. This will include trimming off excess unwanted tissue and cleaning up the blood vessels to the liver ensuring there are no untied branches or defects. It may be necessary to perform reconstructions of the blood vessels if there is anomalous anatomy
- *recipient hepatectomy*: the recipient's diseased liver is dissected free from its peritoneal attachments and adhesions such that it is only left connected by its blood vessels. Clamps are then applied to these vessels and the liver is removed
- *implantation*: the donor liver is taken out of ice and it is implanted in the following sequence:
  – suprahepatic cava
  – infrahepatic cava
  – portal vein: just before completion of the anastomosis the preservation fluid from the donor liver, which has a high potassium content, is flushed out. The anastomosis is then completed and the caval clamps and portal venous clamps are removed to allow reperfusion of the liver
  – arterial anastomosis between the arterial inflow to the liver and the recipient arterial blood flow
  – biliary reconstruction either between the donor and recipient common bile duct or the donor bile duct to a Roux-en-Y loop of small bowel (choledochojejunostomy).

 Vascular complications
- *Haemorrhage* from any of the anastomoses or untied blood vessels or raw surfaces. This would be exacerbated by a coagulopathy as the newly transplanted liver could be inadequate at making clotting factors.
- *Thrombosis/stenosis*: this can occur at any of the anastomoses.
- *Pseudoaneurysms/rupture*: these typically occur at the site of the arterial anastomosis, which has the highest pressure.
- *Hepatic arterial inflow*: the incidence of hepatic artery thrombosis is 1.6–8% and it can be diagnosed in the patient with hepatic dysfunction using duplex ultrasound, and confirmed by angiography. The management if the diagnosis is caught early is by thrombectomy and revision of the anastomosis. Unfortunately if this fails then the patient should be listed for a re-transplant. A stenosis however could be managed by angioplasty.

- *Portal vein inflow*: the incidence of this is approximately 2%, and the patient may present with features of portal hypertension (oesophageal varices, gastrointestinal bleeding and ascites). The diagnosis can be made by Doppler, late-phase arteriography or MRI. The management could be by balloon dilatation with stenting using a 'TIPSS' (transjugular intrahepatic portosystemic shunt). Alternatively surgery could be considered, with an attempt at thrombectomy and revision of the anastomosis.
- *Hepatic vein/inferior vena cava stenosis or thrombosis* of the anastomoses can occur. The patient may present with abdominal pain, ascites, hepatomegaly and bilateral leg oedema. The diagnosis can be suggested on Doppler ultrasound but confirmed using interventional radiological techniques (hepatic or inferior venal cavography). This will allow trans-anastomotic pressure gradients to be measured using a pressure transducer, and the benefit of balloon dilatation can also be determined using this technique.

Biliary tract complications
- These can occur in up to 30% of cases after liver transplants. The biliary tract is critically dependent on the hepatic arterial inflow. The complications that can occur are biliary leaks, strictures (which can be anastomotic or non-anastomotic) and choledocholithiasis (where the stasis of bile flow, for example secondary to a perihilar collection, may give rise to gallstones) or cholangitis.
- The diagnosis can be made by ultrasound to demonstrate intrahepatic biliary duct dilatation and confirm an arterial trace. Any perihilar collections suggestive of a biliary leak can also be demonstrated. An MRCP is also very sensitive at detecting biliary stenoses. In the case of anastomotic biliary stricture, the anastomosis could be dilated with or without the use of a stent using ERCP or PTC. Multiple non-anastomotic strictures however suggest an ischaemic component, and unless this is improved then the patient will be prone to developing multiple abscesses. Often this may be an indication of hepatic artery thrombosis and the patient will need to be considered for a re-transplant. If dilatation fails or the patient is susceptible to recurrent bouts of cholangitis, then a biliary reconstruction using a Roux-en-Y loop should be performed.

Rejection
- *Acute rejection*: there is a 25% risk of acute rejection following liver transplantation. This usually can be treated with steroids.
- *Chronic rejection*: this occurs in approximately 2% of liver transplants, and can occur after the first two months. The management for this is ultimately a new liver transplant.

Recurrence of the original liver disease
It is possible that recurrent disease can occur, and patients should be counselled for this. In some cases this is inevitable such as in hepatitis C, but in other cases prophylaxis can be used (for example hepatitis B). Recurrence can be unpredictable in autoimmune conditions such as primary biliary cirrhosis and primary sclerosing cholangitis. Recurrent or metastatic tumour can occur in cases of transplantation for malignant disease.

Complications of immunosuppression
There are many different immunosuppression drugs and regimes that can be used post-liver transplant. Some of the more frequently observed complications are:
- susceptibility to infections: this includes not only the common hospital-acquired infections but other infections which would not normally cause a significant morbidity in the immunocompetent host. CMV is one example which may cause symptoms of flu

in the immunocompetent host, but in the immunocompromised it could cause a significant disease with:
– oesophagitis
– colitis
– pneumonitis
– meningoencephalitis
– hepatitis
– renal tubulitis
– chorioretinitis
- nephrotoxicity
- higher risk of developing malignancy. As most tumours are virally driven there is an increased susceptibility to nearly all tumours, in particular skin malignancies and lymphoma (post-transplant lymphoproliferative disease)
- diabetes mellitus.

Renal transplant with ureteric obstruction

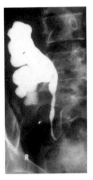

Figure 3.23

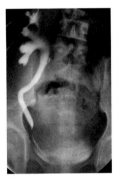

Figure 3.24

Questions

Q1 What is this investigation and what is the diagnosis?

Q2 Describe the radiological features of this investigation.

Q3 How is the diagnosis confirmed?

Q4 What are the causes of this abnormality?

Q5 How should the condition be managed?

Answers

A1 This is an intravenous pyelogram and it demonstrates ureteric obstruction.

A2 There is pelvicalyceal dilatation ('clubbing of the calyces') with dilatation of the ureter, which then comes to a stenotic segment probably at the vesico-ureteric junction. This is not a complete occlusion, as there is some contrast passing into the bladder.

A3
- The patient will present with impairment of renal function from the graft. The obstruction may be painless due to denervation of the graft.
- An ultrasound will demonstrate hydronephrosis although a mild degree of pelvicalyceal dilatation is often seen in renal transplant kidneys.
- An IVP as demonstrated may help confirm the obstruction as well as the site of obstruction, although good visualisation is dependent on reasonable graft function, and the contrast itself can cause a nephropathy.
- A retrograde ureterogram could be attempted but it is difficult to cannulate the transplant ureteral orifice.
- The most reliable means to confirm the diagnosis is by percutaneous antegrade pyelography. This also has the benefit of decompressing the obstruction and allowing recovery of the renal function, while planning a definitive procedure.

A4 The causes can be divided into intraluminal, within the wall of the ureter, and outside the ureter.

Intraluminal
- Blood clots.
- Poor surgical implantation.
- Ureteral slough.
- Ureteral calculus.

Within the wall of the ureter
- Ureteral fibrosis secondary to ischaemia: the ureter receives arterial blood from the main renal artery and during the retrieval process this branch could be damaged, especially if the ureter has been skeletonised from its surrounding peri-ureteric fat.
- Ureteral fibrosis secondary to rejection: if the kidney is rejected, then the ureter may sustain an acute inflammatory injury resulting in fibrosis.
- Infection with polyoma BK virus is a rare cause of ureteric obstruction.

Outside the ureter
- The ureter could be compressed by kinking or twisting. It can also be compressed by haematoma, lymphocoeles and tumours.

A5
- Acute post-operative obstruction usually requires surgical repair. Most centres use a double J-stent to cover the procedure during the peri- and early post-operative period. These are usually removed at 8 weeks. It may be that any abnormality is observed only after this point.
- If the stricture is less than 2 cm long then it may be amenable to endourological techniques in an antegrade or retrograde approach. The stricture can be dilated with a balloon and then under direct vision the stricture can be incised with a cold knife. A stent can then be left in place for 2–6 weeks before being removed cystoscopically.

- If the stricture is more than 2 cm then this will be less amenable to percutaneous techniques and these strictures will require surgical repair (as well as those that fail endourological techniques). This will involve direct implantation of the ureter above the stricture into the bladder or if the stricture is too high then anastomosing the native ureter or bladder to the transplant renal pelvis. To facilitate the latter technique, a psoas hitch could be employed where the bladder wall is sutured to the ipsilateral psoas to reduce tension on the anastomosis. Alternatively a Boari flap could be performed where the bladder is opened with a rectangular incision (preserving one short side) to form a flap, which can be rolled to form a tube and anastomosed to the transplant renal pelvis.

Your revision notes:

Immunological principles of organ transplantation

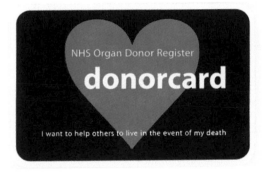

Figure 3.25

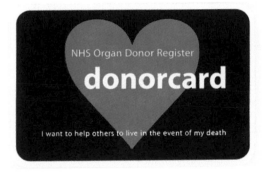

NHS Organ Donor Register

donorcard

I want to help others to live in the event of my death

Figure 3.26

Questions

Q1   What are the different types of grafts?

Q2   What are the immune factors important during transplantation?

Q3   What are the different types of graft rejection?

Q4   What are the ways of preventing graft rejection?

Q5   What are the complications following organ transplantation?

Answers

 • An *allograft* is a graft between two genetically dissimilar individuals of the same species. This was previously called a *homograft*.
• An *isograft* or *syngenic graft* is a graft between two genetically identical individuals of the same species.
• An *autograft* is a graft originating from and applied to the same individual.
• A *xenograft* is a graft between two individuals belonging to two different species.

 • *The ABO blood group barrier*: organ allografts must be ABO compatible but Rhesus testing is not necessary.
• *The major histocompatibility complex*: MHC is a region of the mammalian genome which codes for proteins that have an important role in immunity and are known as transplant antigens. These are encoded by genes in two regions called Class I and Class II regions.
• *Human leucocyte antigen*: HLA comprises two classes (Class1 and Class 2) of cell surface proteins whose principal function is to display peptide antigens so they can be recognised by T cells. The HLA complex is the most polymorphic region of the human genome and is located on the short arm of chromosome 6. The genes within the HLA are divided into three regions known as Class 1, Class 2 and Class 3. Genes in Class 1 encode for HLA-A, HLA-B and HLA-C. These are known as the Classic Class 1 MHC antigens. The non-classic Class 1 MHC antigens are HLA-E, HLA-F and HLA-G. The Class 2 antigens are HLA-DR, HLA-DP and HLA-DQ. The Class 3 antigens are not major transplant antigens.

 • *Hyperacute rejection*: this occurs within minutes or hours of transplantation and is due to preformed antibodies in the recipient. There is extensive intravascular thrombosis seen.
• *Acute rejection*: this occurs within days to weeks of transplantation. It is not usually encountered beyond the first six months. It is usually associated with progressive mononuclear cell infiltratin of the graft due to cellular effector mechanisms.
• *Chronic rejection*: this usually occurs beyond the first six months. There is progressive myointimal proliferation within the arteries of the graft leading to ischaemia. Both alloantibodies and cellular effector mechanisms are thought to play a part.

 ABO blood group compatibility, antibody screening, HLA typing, immunosuppressive therapy using steroids, cyclosporin, tacrolimus, azathioprine, sirolimus, polyclonal anti-lymphocyte antibodies, OKT3, IL-2 receptor antibodies.

(A5) • Infections: bacterial, e.g. *Pneumocystis carinii*; viral, e.g. CMV, Herpes, EBV; fungal, e.g. *Candida*, *Aspergillus*.
• Malignancies, e.g. lymphomas, skin cancers, urogenital cancers, Kaposi's sarcoma.
• Rejection.
• Specific problems associated with different transplant operations.

Section 4

Paediatric surgery

Spina bifida

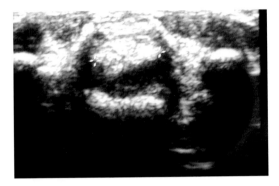

Figure 4.1

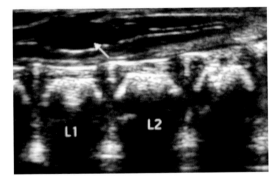

Figure 4.2

This neonate was brought after the discovery of a soft lump over the lower back midline. The lump resembled a lipoma clinically, and an ultrasound of the area (Figure 4.1) confirmed this with an underlying spina bifida.

Questions

Q1 What is spina bifida?

Q2 What is spina bifida occulta? How do you suspect this?

Q3 What is a meningocoele (see Figure 4.2)?

Q4 What is a myelomeningocoele?

Q5 What are the aetiological factors for this abnormality?

Q6 What are the associated abnormalities?

Q7 What are the possible neurological sequelae?

Q8 How is it managed?

Answers

A1 It is a developmental defect of the posterior vertebral arch resulting in the absence of spinous processes and variable amounts of laminae.

A2 Spina bifida occulta is not associated with meningeal protrusion and can be an incidental and asymptomatic radiological finding. Overlying cutaneous stigmata such as a lipoma, port wine stain, tuft of hair or a dimple may be present. Direct spinal cord compression or tethering can sometimes cause neurological symptoms.

A3 Protrusion of the meningeal coverings through the spinal column is termed meningocoele. This clinically presents as a soft, reducible and pedunculated mass, which demonstrates trans-illumination. The underlying spinal cord is normal and hence this is not associated with neurological problems. Rupture and secondary infection can, however, cause problems. The treatment is aimed at decompression, closure of the CSF fistula and release of the spinal cord tethering.

A4 Myelomeningocoele is the protrusion of nervous tissue along with the meningeal coverings. This is the most important spinal dysgraphic disorder with an incidence of 1–2 per 1000 live births. Effective prenatal screening (maternal AFP) has reduced the incidence. There is an ethnic variation with more cases in the British Isles and in those of Celtic origin and less in Asians.

A5 The aetiological factors are multifactorial and heterogeneous. Chromosomal abnormalities, gene mutations, drugs (e.g. carbamazepine, valproic acid), environmental factors such as famine, poverty and maternal folate deficiency have been thought to play a role.

A6 The associated abnormalities are: Arnold–Chiari malformation (prolongation of the medulla, tonsils and cerebellar vermis through the foramen magnum) resulting in hydrocephalus and vertebral anomalies such as kyphosis and kyphoscoliosis.

A7 The neurological sequelae may include motor loss, sensory loss or autonomic involvement. Lesions below T12 are associated with complete paraplegia. Autonomic dysfunction will lead to neurogenic bladder and bowel incontinence.

A8 Management involves a multidisciplinary approach by a team, which includes neonatologists, neurosurgeons, physiotherapists, paediatric and orthopaedic surgeons. Nursing in the prone position, antibiotics if there is rupture of the sac, and bladder catheterisation are common requirements. Surgery is aimed at preserving neurological function and prevention of CSF leak. With modern treatments about 85% survive with varying degrees of disability.

Intussusception

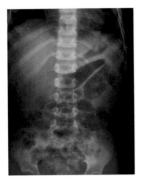

Figure 4.3

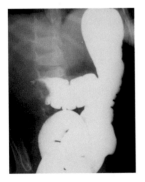

Figure 4.4

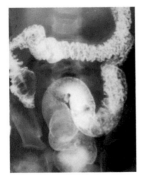

Figure 4.5

An eight-month-old infant was brought with a history of episodes of abdominal pain associated with passage of blood stained stools. The AXR (Figure 4.3) and barium enema films (Figures 4.4 and 4.5) are shown.

Questions

Q1 What do the AXR and barium enema films show?

Q2 What is the diagnosis? What is the usual area involved?

Q3 What is the usual age group affected? What are the suspected risk factors?

Q4 What is the typical clinical presentation?

Q5 What is the 'sign de Dance'?

Q6 How is the diagnosis confirmed?

Q7 What is the treatment?

Q8 What are the indications for operative management?

Answers

(A1) The plain AXR (Figure 4.3) shows signs of small bowel obstruction. Figure 4.4 shows the typical 'claw sign', and Figure 4.5 is a barium enema after hydrostatic reduction.

(A2) Intussusception is the telescoping of one portion of the intestine into another. It is the most common cause of intestinal obstruction in early childhood. The usual location is the ileo-caecal area.

(A3) The most common age group is the infant between 6 and 9 months. Several factors have been suggested such as changes in diet and lymphoid hyperplasia. In the older child it can be secondary to other causes such as Meckel's diverticulum, appendix, intestinal neoplasm, submucosal haemorrhage (Henoch–Schönlein purpura), foreign body, ectopic pancreatic or gastric tissue and intestinal duplication.

(A4) This classically produces severe crampy abdominal pain in an otherwise healthy child. The child often draws up his/her legs during the episodes and is quite withdrawn in between episodes. Vomiting is almost always present. Frequent bowel movement leading to the passage of 'redcurrant jelly'-like stools may occur. A sausage-shaped mass may be palpable.

(A5) The right iliac fossa normally occupied by the caecum may appear quite empty and is called the 'sign de Dance'.

(A6) The diagnosis can be suspected in half of the cases on the plain AXR. An abdominal ultrasound may show characteristic findings of a 'target lesion' or a 'pseudo kidney' appearance on longitudinal section. A contrast enema is diagnostic ('claw sign') and can also be therapeutic. Contraindications to the enema include the presence of peritonitis and haemodynamic instability.

(A7) Hydrostatic reduction using barium or even air has been the mainstay of therapy. Successful reduction can occur in 80% of cases. Saline enema under ultrasound guidance can avoid radiation exposure. The recurrence rate after hydrostatic reduction is about 10% and usually occurs within the first 24 h. The recurrence is usually managed by a repeat hydrostatic reduction with surgery reserved for those with a third occurrence.

(A8) The usual indications for surgery are peritonitis, clinical suspicion of necrotic bowel, complete small bowel obstruction, failure of hydrostatic reduction and history of several recurrences. An initial laparoscopic approach can be tried. Careful examination of the bowel is mandatory after reduction. Adhesive bands around the ileo-caecal area are divided and appendicectomy performed. Indications for bowel resection include failure to reduce the intussusception, concerns about bowel viability and finding a lead-point for the intussusception.

Duodenal atresia

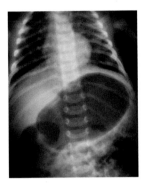

Figure 4.6

A one-week-old infant is brought with a history of inability to tolerate feeds and persistent vomiting since birth. The vomitus is bilious in nature. The AXR taken to investigate this is shown in Figure 4.6.

Questions

Q1 What is the diagnosis? What are the causes?

Q2 How do you confirm the diagnosis?

Q3 How is this condition treated?

Q4 How do you differentiate this condition from pyloric stenosis?

Answers

(A1) Duodenal atresia (DA). This results from a failure of vacuolisation of the duodenum from its solid cord stage. The range of anatomical variants includes duodenal stenosis, mucosal web with intact muscular wall ('windsock deformity'), the two ends separated by a fibrous cord and a complete separation with a gap in between. The associated conditions include Down's syndrome, maternal polyhydramnios, malrotation of the gut, annular pancreas and biliary atresia. Cardiac, renal, oesophageal and anorectal malformations may also be present.

(A2) The classic plain AXR sign is a 'double bubble appearance' (air-filled stomach and duodenal bulb). Upper GI contrast studies are sometimes required if distal air is present.

(A3) The treatment of DA is by surgical bypass by a side-to-side duodeno-duodenostomy. A tapering duodenoplasty of the proximal duodenum is sometimes needed to reduce the calibre if it is hugely dilated.

(A4) The clinical presentation is similar to hypertrophic pyloric stenosis but can be differentiated by bilious vomiting, absence of a palpable 'pyloric tumour' and the double bubble sign.

Infantile hypertrophic pyloric stenosis

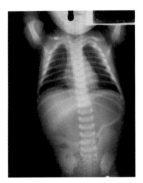

Figure 4.7

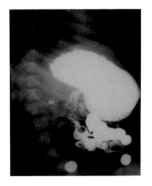

Figure 4.10

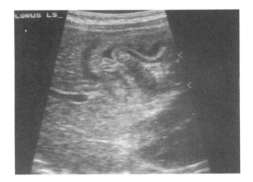

Figure 4.8

A 4-week-old male infant was brought with a history of persistent vomiting and losing weight. The findings on the AXR (Figure 4.7), ultrasound scans (Figures 4.8 and 4.9) and barium meal (Figure 4.10) are shown.

Questions

Q1 What are the findings on the AXR, ultrasound and barium meal? What is this condition and what is its incidence?

Q2 What is the underlying abnormality?

Q3 What are the clinical features?

Q4 How do you diagnose this?

Q5 What are the typical metabolic changes associated with this?

Q6 How do you treat this? What are the potential complications?

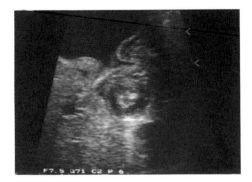

Figure 4.9

Answers

A1
- The AXR shows gas in a hugely distended stomach. The barium meal confirms a distended stomach with narrowing of the pylorus causing obstruction of the gastric outlet. The ultrasound also shows a grossly thickened pylorus, which displays the 'target sign' on cross-section.
- The diagnosis is hypertrophic pyloric stenosis of infancy. The incidence is approximately 3–4 per 1000 live births. It is four to five times more common in male infants. The cause is unknown, but multiple factors have been suggested. Ethnicity may be an important factor as it is more common in Scandinavian individuals of white descent and least common in African-Americans and Chinese. There is a higher risk in the offspring of patients and it frequently affects the first-born males.

A2
The underlying pathology is hypertrophy of the circular muscle of the pylorus and the adjacent antrum, which results in constriction and obstruction of the gastric outlet. The hypertrophy is maximal in the pylorus. The mucosa is compressed and a probe is only inserted with difficulty.

A3
The condition is most commonly seen about 3–4 weeks after birth. The typical symptom is vomiting which becomes forcible and projectile. The vomitus does not contain bile. The baby is usually hungry. Weight loss is striking and the baby becomes emaciated and dehydrated. Stools are hard and infrequent.

A4
Clinical diagnosis is by finding the typical wave of peristalsis in the upper abdomen with palpation of the olive-shaped 'pyloric tumour'. Diagnosis is made by a test feed. Ultrasound is the investigation of choice and shows the hypertrophied muscle as a broad ring with low echo density while the mucosa appears as an inner layer of high echo density. In doubtful cases a barium contrast study will show gastric outlet obstruction with a narrowed pylorus.

A5
Low sodium chloride, low potassium, metabolic alkalosis, dehydration, nutritional emaciation. Renal compensation occurs to substitute K^+ for Na^+.

A6
- The first concern is to treat the metabolic abnormalities. The infant should be rehydrated with dextrose–saline and potassium (2.5% dextrose plus 0.45% sodium chloride plus 1 g KCl per 500 ml fluid).
- Surgical correction is then planned. The name of the operation is Ramstedt's operation (after the German surgeon Wilhelm Conrad Ramstedt who performed this in 1911). This consists of a pyloromyotomy to divide the hypertrophied pyloric muscle. The operation can be done under either local or general anaesthesia. An upper abdominal transverse incision is made overlying the palpable pyloric lump. The muscle has the consistency of an unripened pear and the mucosa bulges out after the division of muscle is complete. Care should be taken not to penetrate the mucosa. If this happens, it is closed with a piece of omentum.
- Wound infection occurs in about 5% of infants, and 1% will suffer wound disruption (more common in emaciated infants).

Undescended testis

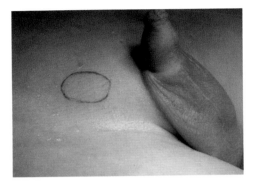

Figure 4.11

A 2-year-old boy is about to undergo surgery following an observation made on his genitalia and a lump in his right groin (Figure 4.11).

Questions

Q1 What is the most likely diagnosis?

Q2 What is the differential diagnosis?

Q3 Can these conditions be distinguished clinically?

Q4 Where is the right testis lying in this case and how do you know that it is not within the inguinal canal?

Q5 What are the complications of this condition?

Q6 Figure 4.12 shows the completed operation on another patient. What has been performed?

Q7 Are there any useful investigations to perform prior to surgery? Does the fact that the testis is ectopic (not in the normal line of descent) rather than maldescended change your management?

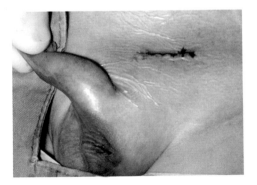

Figure 4.12

Answers

(A1) Undescended testis/ectopic testis.

(A2) The differential diagnosis is a retractile testis.

(A3) A retractile testis is a normal testicle where an excessively active cremasteric reflex draws the testis up to the superficial inguinal ring. On careful examination in a warm atmosphere it can be coaxed into the scrotum. An ectopic testis cannot be manipulated into the scrotum. If the testis is retractile, the scrotum is normally developed. No further intervention is required. The testicle is likely to descend normally by puberty. Follow-up is mandatory.

(A4) The testis is easily visible and therefore is lying in the superficial inguinal pouch having emerged from the external ring. If it were still lying within the inguinal canal, it would not be certainly visible and probably not palpable.

(A5) Complications of this condition include:
- defective spermatogenesis – sterility if bilateral
- increased risk of torsion
- increased risk of trauma
- inguinal herniation (associated in 90%)
- increased risk of malignant change (relative risk of 20–40%), which appears to be the case even if surgical correction is performed.

(A6)
- Orchidopexy: mobilisation and placement of the testis into the scrotum. This should be carried out as soon as possible. Remember '2 in the bag by the age of 2'! The co-existing inguinal hernia sac should be removed at the same time.
- Exploration is via a high inguinal incision allowing first the inguinal canal then the abdominal cavity to be explored.

(A7)
- Since surgery is always indicated, investigations such as USS (unreliable), MRI and CT (needs anaesthetic) and laparoscopy (normally leads to open surgery) are not indicated.
- Management is as for undescended testis. If a testis is located and found to be dysplastic it must be removed. If normal it must be replaced into the scrotum. There is no indication for testicular biopsy.

Diaphragmatic hernia

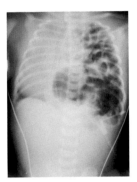

Figure 4.13

This neonate had respiratory distress soon after birth.

Questions

Q1 What does the CXR show? What is the diagnosis?

Q2 What is the commonest site? What are the other sites?

Q3 What are the clinical features seen?

Q4 How is the diagnosis confirmed?

Q5 How is this condition treated?

Q6 What is the prognosis?

Answers

(A1) The CXR shows bowel loops within the chest cavity. The diagnosis is a diaphragmatic hernia. The incidence is approximately 1 in 3500 live births; 80% of these occur on the left side.

(A2) The commonest type is in the postero-lateral situation through the foramen of Bochdalek. This foramen is the result of failure of closure of the pleuroperitoneal canal. The other types are through the foramen of Morgagni, hiatus, dome and central tendon.

(A3) The typical presentation is with respiratory difficulty starting soon after birth. The classic triad of signs is respiratory distress/cyanosis, mediastinal shift (apparent dextrocardia) and a scaphoid abdomen.

(A4) The diagnosis is frequently made during a routine antenatal ultrasound examination. A CXR after birth confirms the diagnosis.

(A5) Early placement of a nasogastric tube will help to prevent bowel distension in the chest. Ventilation and correction of acid–base abnormalities may sometimes be necessary before surgical intervention. The definitive treatment is an operation to reduce the hernial contents and repair the defect. This is usually done through a subcostal abdominal incision. Prosthetic material may be used if there is not sufficient diaphragm available.

(A6) The overall mortality is around 40–50% and depends on residual lung volume and function.

Hypospadias

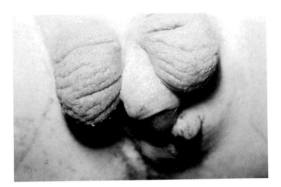

Figure 4.14

Questions

Q1 What is the diagnosis?

Q2 What has failed during development?

Q3 What are the principle components of this condition?

Q4 How do you classify this condition?

Q5 What is important to establish on presentation?

Q6 What is the treatment? What are the potential complications?

Answers

A1 Hypospadias: a common anomalous development of the distal urethra, penile shaft and glans penis affecting 1 in 400 boys.

A2 The male urethra is formed by the in-rolling of the genital folds. In hypospadias the urethral plate and groove fail to complete the process of tubularisation and fusion.

A3
- The urethra opens onto the ventral surface anywhere from the glans to perineum.
- Ventral curvature (chordee) of the penile shaft due to the presence of fibrous tissue within the penile fascia.
- Deficient ventral foreskin and excess hooded dorsal foreskin.

A4 It can involve the glans alone or any degree of the penile and perineal urethra. Classification is as follows:
- glanular
- distal/mid/proximal penile
- scrotal
- perineal (15%).

The more proximal position of the urethral orifice makes surgery more difficult and complex.

A5 On presentation it is important to establish whether hypospadias is an isolated anomaly or whether other urinary tract anomalies co-exist. This is unusual with the more usual glanular/distal penile cases. With more proximal abnormalities, associated anomalies need to be excluded with ultrasound. Other common anomalies in this condition are inguinal hernias and an undescended testis.

A6 Treatment depends on the site of urethral orifice:
- glanular hypospadias: meatal advancement and glanuloplasty (MAGPI). This can be done as a day case procedure and does not require catheter drainage
- more complex problems may require onlay graft and island flap urethroplasty involving release of the chordee and construction of a neourethra using imported tissue.

Potential complications of surgery are:
- skin ischaemia
- haematoma formation
- infection
- fistula formation
- urethral stenosis
- residual chordee.

Foreign body

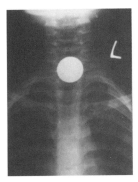

Figure 4.15

Figure 4.15 shows an X-ray of a young boy who presents with sudden onset dysphagia and neck discomfort.

Questions

Q1   What is the diagnosis?

Q2   What are the usual clinical symptoms? What is the usual site of lodgement?

Q3   What are the usual objects involved?

Q4   What are the clinical findings?

Q5   How do you treat this problem?

Answers

(A1) A foreign body in the upper oesophagus.

(A2) Patients usually present with pain in the neck or chest, increased salivation, and dysphagia. The foreign body usually lodges at the narrowest point of the upper GI tract, i.e. the post-cricoid region of the cricopharyngeus muscle.

(A3) The most common object involved in children is a coin. In adults, bone, false teeth and food bolus are common. Various objects can be encountered in psychiatric patients, e.g. razors and batteries. Ingested drug packets are also encountered.

(A4) Examination can be completely normal. However the patient is usually drooling. Surgical emphysema can be rarely present. X-rays reveal the radio-opaque foreign bodies. Oesophageal air bubble or soft tissue swelling can occasionally be seen.

(A5)
- Soft foreign bodies, e.g. meat bolus not containing bone, may be managed medically with a combination of muscle relaxants and an anti-inflammatory agent. Giving aerated drinks such as Coke can sometimes help.
- The foreign bodies that do not respond to this will require flexible (or rigid) oesophago-gastroscopy under sedation, and removal. A bolus is sometimes removed piecemeal or pushed into the stomach. A patient with bolus impaction should undergo contrast swallow studies later on to rule out strictures.
- A patient with a history of a sharp foreign body should not be given muscle relaxants or anti-inflammatory drugs as they may cause perforation. These patients will require rigid endoscopy and the foreign body should be retrieved into the scope and the whole apparatus removed *en bloc*. The oesophagus is reassessed after this. Following this the patient needs to be nil by mouth for 2–4 h, and a watch kept for possible oesophageal perforation.

Exomphalos

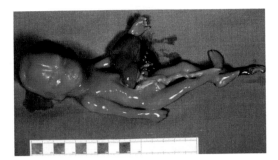

Figure 4.16

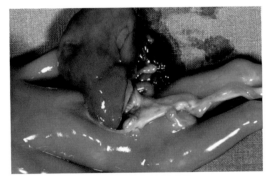

Figure 4.17

Questions

Q1 What is the diagnosis?

Q2 What is the underlying pathogenesis?

Q3 What types are there and what is the incidence?

Q4 What is gastroschisis? How may the two conditions be distinguished?

Q5 What are the principles of management of an exomphalos?

Q6 What is the prognosis?

Answers

(A1)   Exomphalos.

(A2)   The underlying pathogenesis is failure of rotation and return of all or part of the mid-gut into the abdominal cavity during fetal life. This occurs through an abdominal wall defect greater than 4 cm in size. A defect of less than 4 cm is referred to as a hernia of the umbilical cord.

(A3)   There are two types:
- *major:* partial or total persistence of mid-gut within the umbilical cord
- *minor:* the herniation of one or two bowel loops into the base of the umbilical cord. Incidence is 1:4000 live births.

(A4)
- Gastroschisis is a full-thickness abdominal wall defect in which there is herniation of uncovered bowel loops (there are no coverings).
- An exomphalos is covered with a sac consisting of fetal membranes, and the umbilical cord inserts centrally over the defect. A gastroschisis is not covered by a sac and the herniation occurs to the right of the umbilical cord.
- Exomphalos is associated with other congenital abnormalities (50% incidence) including neurological, cardiac, chromosomal and gastrointestinal (Meckel's diverticulum and intestinal atresia) abnormalities.
- Gastroschisis is rarely associated with other anomalies but there is ~15% incidence of atresias secondary to pressure ischaemia at the neck of the defect.

(A5)
- Immediate surgical repair should be carried out if possible.
- The viscera should be kept warm and moist with a dressing soaked in mild antiseptic (usually silver sulphadiazine). This should then be packed in a plastic drape to avoid evaporation.
- The patient should be on intravenous antibiotics to avoid sepsis.
- The main aim is to return the viscera into the abdominal cavity. If the abdominal cavity cannot contain the viscera, a polypropylene mesh can be used with gradual closure of the abdomen over a period of days. Gradual epithelialisation and slow reduction take place as well, and in minor exomphalos you can await spontaneous closure.
- Total parenteral nutrition is often needed until the gut starts to function.

(A6)
- Overall outcome depends on the presence and severity of associated abnormalities.
- Infection and pulmonary insufficiency are significant risks, and survival from major exomphalos is around 50% despite intensive supportive therapy.

Hirschsprung's disease

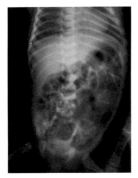

Figure 4.18

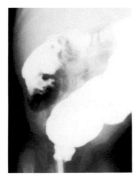

Figure 4.19

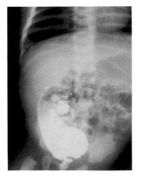

Figure 4.20

This neonate was brought with a history of delayed passage of meconium followed by ongoing constipation and abdominal distension. The AXR (Figure 4.18) and barium enema (Figures 4.19 and 4.20) performed are shown.

Questions

Q1 What is the diagnosis? What is the underlying abnormality?

Q2 What are the different clinical presentations?

Q3 How is the diagnosis confirmed?

Q4 What are the different described surgical options? What is the most common post-operative problem?

Answers

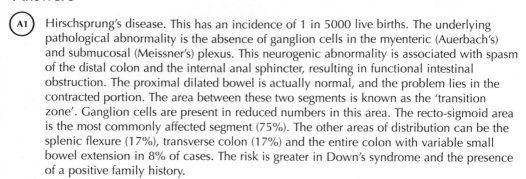

A1 Hirschsprung's disease. This has an incidence of 1 in 5000 live births. The underlying pathological abnormality is the absence of ganglion cells in the myenteric (Auerbach's) and submucosal (Meissner's) plexus. This neurogenic abnormality is associated with spasm of the distal colon and the internal anal sphincter, resulting in functional intestinal obstruction. The proximal dilated bowel is actually normal, and the problem lies in the contracted portion. The area between these two segments is known as the 'transition zone'. Ganglion cells are present in reduced numbers in this area. The recto-sigmoid area is the most commonly affected segment (75%). The other areas of distribution can be the splenic flexure (17%), transverse colon (17%) and the entire colon with variable small bowel extension in 8% of cases. The risk is greater in Down's syndrome and the presence of a positive family history.

A2 Most cases are symptomatic within the first 24 h of life, with progressive abdominal distension and bilious vomiting. Failure to pass meconium is a cardinal feature of this condition. Diarrhoea can sometimes be seen due to enterocolitis. Some cases present later in older children with a history of poor feeding, chronic abdominal distension and chronic constipation.

A3 The initial diagnostic step is a plain AXR (showing large bowel obstruction) followed by a barium enema. Rectal examination prior to this should be avoided to prevent interfering with locating the transition zone. The two common findings on a barium enema would be a rectum with a smaller calibre than the sigmoid colon, and failure to completely evacuate the barium even after 24 h. Anorectal manometry can help in diagnosis and the classic finding is failure of the internal sphincter to relax when the rectum is distended with a balloon (recto-anal inhibitory reflex). Rectal biopsy is the gold standard in the diagnosis. The sample is obtained from at least 2 cm from the dentate line.

A4 • Multiple surgical options are available for the management of Hirschsprung's disease. It is usually managed by an initial defunctioning stoma followed later by one of the following three definitive procedures:
  – *Duhamel's procedure*: the aganglionic rectal stump is left in place and the ganglionated normal colon is pulled behind this and a GIA stapler used to create a colo-anal anastomosis and a neorectum
  – *Svenson's procedure*: the aganglionic segment is removed up to the level of the internal sphincters, and a colo-anal anastomosis performed on the perineum
  – *Soave procedure*: an endo-rectal mucosal dissection within the aganglionic distal rectum is done. The normal colon is pulled through the remnant muscular cuff and a colo-anal anastomosis performed.
• The overall survival in this condition is excellent. Constipation is the most frequent post-operative problem. Soiling and incontinence may also be seen.

Section 5

Breast and

endocrine surgery

Breast cancer (1)

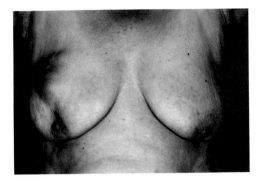

Figure 5.1

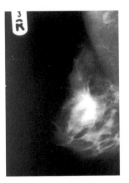

Figure 5.2

A 59-year-old lady presented with a two-week history of noticing this painless lump in her right breast (Figure 5.1).

Questions

Q1 Describe three features of the abnormality seen.

Q2 What is triple assessment?

Q3 Describe the features of malignancy on a mammogram (Figure 5.2).

Q4 Is breast conservation surgery an option? Why/Why not?

Q5 What is the Nottingham Prognostic Index (NPI)?

Answers

1 A large irregular mass in the upper quadrant of the right breast.
2 Skin dimpling.
3 Retraction of the nipple.
These are typical features of a breast carcinoma. Typically on inspection, a large mass, skin tethering, nipple tethering, nipple inversion, peau d'orange are seen. On palpation, there is a well-defined, irregular, hard, fixed or mobile mass.

1 Clinical examination.
2 Mammogram +/– ultrasound of the breast.
3 Fine needle aspiration cytology/core biopsy.
The triple assessment is a truly multidisciplinary approach involving the clinician, radiologist and the pathologist.

- A spiculated mass.
- Abnormal microcalcifications.
- Architectural distortion or stellate lesions.
- Asymmetry.
A spiculated mass is a definable central mass with irregular margins and distortion of the surrounding tissue. Microcalcifications within and around the tumour mass are typically associated with ductal carcinoma *in situ* (DCIS). Ultrasound of the breast typically shows an irregular mass of low and mixed echogenicity with distal acoustic shadowing.

Breast conservation surgery (BCS) is not an option as the tumour is relatively large, associated with skin involvement. The most appropriate operation is mastectomy with level 3 axillary clearance. Factors favouring mastectomy over BCS are:
- large size of the primary compared to the size of the breast
- central location of the tumour
- multifocal tumour
- patient desire
- age of the patient: older patients prefer mastectomy compared to younger women, who opt for BCS.

The NPI is a combination of three factors to identify the prognosis of the tumour:
1 tumour size
2 tumour grade
3 presence and level of histological nodal involvement (stage).
It is calculated by the following formula:
Grade + LN + (tumour size in cm × 0.2)
- *Tumour grade*: is measured by the pathologist by Elston's method which scores mitosis, pleomorphism and tubule formation:
  – 1 = well differentiated
  – 2 = moderately differentiated
  – 3 = poorly differentiated.
- *Lymph nodes* (stage, LN) are measured from 1 to 3:
  – no nodes = 1
  – 1–3 nodes involved = 2
  – 4 or more nodes or high lymph node = 3.
- *Tumour size*: measured on histology (maximum diameter in cm).
- *Prognostic value*:
  – <3.4 = excellent (15 year survival ~90%)
  – 3.4–5.4 = moderate
  – >5.4 poor.

Breast cancer (2)

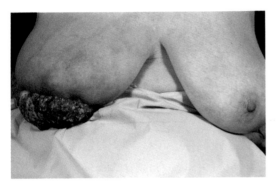

Figure 5.3

A 68-year-old lady presented in clinic with this breast lesion.

Questions

Q1   What is the diagnosis?

Q2   What are the risk factors for developing this condition?

Q3   How do we investigate this lesion?

Q4   How do we stage this lesion?

Q5   What are the treatment options?

Answers

(A1) Fungating carcinoma of the right breast.

(A2) Carcinoma of the female breast is the most common female cancer. It is the leading cause of death in women between the ages of 40 and 50 years. The aetiology is not known but genetic, endocrine and dietary factors are implicated in its genesis.

Risk factors
- *Age*: linear increase with age so older people are more at risk. ✔
- *Female sex* (remember it can occur in men). ✔
- *Oestrogen exposure*: early menarche, late menopause, oral contraceptive pill. ✔
- *Nulliparous*: early pregnancy is protective, as is multiparity. ✔
- *Previous breast cysts*: 2× risk. ✔
- *Weight*: in patients >55 years. ✔
- *Family history and genetic factors*:
  - *BRCA1* (2% all breast carcinomas) and *BRCA2*: *BRCA1* is located on chromosome 11 and is associated with both breast and ovarian cancer development, whereas *BRCA2* is on chromosome 17 and is associated with breast cancer only
  - *RR5* if multiple relatives affected
  - *RR9* if first-degree relative with bilateral carcinoma
  - Li–Fraumeni syndrome (increased risk of multiple primary cancers).
- *Geography*: high in North America and Europe, low in Africa and SE Asia.
- *Atypical hyperplasia*. ✔
- *Class*: upper class > lower class. ✔
- *Marriage*: unmarried > married. ✔
- *Jews* and *nuns* have higher risk. ✔

(A3) • Biopsy and histology.

(A4) • Chest X-ray. ✔
- CT of the chest, abdomen and pelvis. ✔
- Bone scan. ✔
- CA 15-3. ✔

Staging is done to assess the extent of spread. Breast cancer commonly spreads to the axillary lymph nodes, internal mammary lymph nodes and supraclavicular lymph nodes. Distant metastases are by systemic circulation rather than portal route. The principal site ➜ of metastases is the bone. Other sites are the lungs, liver and brain.

(A5) • Hormonal therapy if the tumour is oestrogen-receptor positive. ✔
- Systemic neo-adjuvant chemotherapy to shrink the tumour before contemplating local surgery or radiotherapy.
- Current treatments have some impact on local control but have had little impact on survival. Patients with hormone-sensitive disease have a much longer survival than those with hormone-insensitive disease. Local and regional relapse occurs in 50% of patients. The mainstay of local treatments has been radiotherapy. Combining systemic therapy and radiotherapy, response rates of over 80% have been reported.
- The prognosis is poor with advanced disease.

Breast cancer (3)

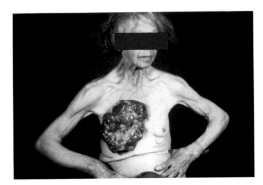

Figure 5.4

A 79-year-old lady presented with this lesion on her anterior chest wall.

Questions

Q1 What is the diagnosis?

Q2 How do you investigate and, ideally, stage this condition?

Q3 Name three staging systems.

Q4 What is the incidence of this condition in males?

Q5 Name three modes of spread of this condition.

Q6 What are ductal carcinoma *in situ* (DCIS) and lobular carcinoma *in situ* (LCIS)?

Answers

(A1) Large fungating carcinoma of the right breast replacing the breast, along with involvement of the chest wall.

(A2) Open biopsy to confirm diagnosis and also the oestrogen-receptor status of the lesion.
Staging
- Chest X-ray.
- CT of the chest, abdomen and pelvis.
- Bone scan.
- CA 15-3.

(A3)
- Union Internationale Contre le Cancer (UICC).
- Manchester.
- Columbia.

All three systems describe the clinical staging of the disease by reference to the primary tumour, regional nodal areas and systemic disease. As the UICC system is more universal and comprehensive it is used more often.

UICC TNM classification
Primary tumour = T

Tx	Not assessable
T0	No primary tumour
TIS	Carcinoma in situ/Paget's disease
T1	2 cm or less
T1a	<0.5 cm
T1b	0.6–1 cm
T1c	1.1–2cm
T2	>2 cm but <5 cm
T3	>5 cm
T4	Any size with chest wall or skin extension
T4a	Chest wall
T4b	Oedema/ulceration/nodules
T4c	Both 4a and 4b
T4d	Inflammatory cancer

Nodes = N

Nx	Not assessable
N0	No node metastasis
N1	Mobile ipsilateral axillary
N2	Fixed ipsilateral axillary
N3	Ipsilateral internal mammary nodes

Distant metastasis = M

Mx	Not assessable
M0	No distant metastasis
M1	Distant metastasis present

(A4) ~1% of all cancers
- Average age in men is 60 years compared to 50 years in a lady.
- The most common symptom is a mass in the breast, however there is delay in seeking advice. In view of the small size of the gland and also delay in presenting, the condition is usually advanced. The treatment for loco-regional disease is radical mastectomy (as, usually, the muscles are involved) and axillary surgery. Systemic adjuvant therapy like tamoxifen can be commenced depending on the histology.

- *Lymphatic*: axillary, internal mammary and supraclavicular lymph nodes.
- *Haematogenous*: lungs, liver, brain, bones.
- *Transcoelomic*: ascites, pleural effusion.

Ductal carcinoma *in situ*

DCIS is a non-invasive precancerous process. It occurs most commonly in the 40–60-year-old age group and presents with a nipple discharge and/or a mass. DCIS is usually unilateral and, if left untreated, proceeds to invasive ductal carcinoma. There is a 25–50% risk of breast cancer at 10–15 years. When DCIS recurs, 50% will be invasive tumours.

Lobular carcinoma *in situ*

LCIS is found predominantly in premenopausal women. It does not present as a mass and is often seen in biopsies. It is often associated with an infiltrating tumour, but not necessarily lobular carcinoma.

Your revision notes:

Cystosarcoma phylloides

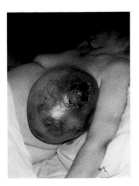

Figure 5.5

Questions

Q1   What is the lesion illustrated in this picture?

Q2   What is the differential diagnosis of this type of lesion?

Q3   What are the typical findings on clinical examination?

Q4   What investigational modalities are available?

Q5   What is the histological appearance?

Q6   What are the treatment modalities?

Answers

(A1) The illustrated lesion is called cystosarcoma phylloides. This is a rare, predominantly benign tumour that occurs almost exclusively in the female breast mainly in the fifth and sixth decades. The name originated from the Greek language where 'sarcoma' means a fleshy tumour and 'phyllo' means a leaf. This name is attributed due to the characteristics of a large malignant sarcoma-like lesion clinically, leaf-like appearance when sectioned, and further display of epithelial cyst-like spaces when viewed histologically. Because most tumours are benign, the name may be misleading. However, these lesions can undergo malignant change and the incidence of malignancy is about 15–30%. Curiously, it is more common on the left side.

(A2)
- Breast cancer.
- Giant fibroadenoma.
- Inflammatory carcinoma.
- Fat necrosis.
- Fibrocystic change.
- Breast abscess.
- Mastitis.
- Angiosarcoma.

(A3) This presents as a firm, mobile, well-circumscribed, non-tender breast mass similar to a fibroadenoma but larger in size. The overlying skin may display a stretched and shiny appearance and be translucent enough that underlying breast veins are visible. They sometimes manifest as a rapid growth. This may be a sign of malignant change. Common metastatic sites include the lungs, skeleton and the liver.

(A4) Mammography and ultrasound findings are similar to fibroadenoma, i.e. round densities with smooth borders. They are hence very unreliable in differentiating the benign from the malignant variants as well as from a fibroadenoma. FNA for cytological examination is usually inadequate for diagnosis. Open excisional breast biopsy is the definitive method to diagnose this lesion.

(A5)
- The content of stromal component can vary significantly among the cystosarcoma phylloides.
- Benign cystosarcoma demonstrate regular fusiform fibroblasts in the stroma. There may be occasional anaplastic cells with myxoid changes.
- Malignant cystosarcoma demonstrate increased atypical cells and increased cellularity of the stroma.

(A6) Surgery:
- in most cases, a wide local excision with a rim of normal tissue
- if the tumour-to-breast ratio is sufficiently high to preclude a satisfactory cosmetic result by segmental excision, total mastectomy, with or without reconstruction, is an alternative
- more radical procedures are not generally warranted
- an axillary lymph node dissection is performed only for clinically suspicious nodes. However, virtually all of these nodes are reactive and do not contain malignant cells
- tumours initially treated by wide local excision that recur locally can be treated by a further wide local excision, but ideally they are treated by total mastectomy.

Response to chemotherapy and radiotherapy for recurrences and metastases has been poor, and no success with hormonal manipulation has been documented.

Gynaecomastia

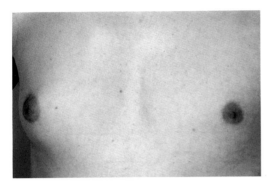

Figure 5.6

A 14-year-old boy was brought in by his mother with this abnormality of 6 months' duration.

Questions

Q1 What is the diagnosis?

Q2 Name two common presenting symptoms.

Q3 Name three causes of this condition.

Q4 What are the treatment options?

Answers

(A1) Unilateral gynaecomastia.

(A2)
- Slowly progressive diffuse swelling.
- Pain and tenderness.

(A3) Causes can be classified as:
- primary or physiological
- secondary.

Primary is classified as:
- *infantile*: usually resolves by four months of age
- *adolescent*: usually idiopathic and resolves in 6 months but may persist for 2 years
- *adult*: may resolve spontaneously.

The commonest secondary causes are drugs, e.g. digoxin, steroids, cimetidine and spironolactone, and high alcohol consumption. Other causes are:
- chronic liver disease
- Addison's disease
- thyrotoxicosis
- testicular, bronchogenic, adrenal tumours
- testicular failure secondary to Klinefelter's syndrome and cryptorchidism.

(A4)
- Reassurance: most men are reassured after malignancy is excluded with imaging.
- Identify and treat secondary causes.
- Stop any relevant medications.
- Surgery (excision of breast with preservation of the nipple) is only indicated if it is very painful or for cosmetic reasons. This is usually in the form of a subcutaneous mastectomy.

Paget's disease of the nipple

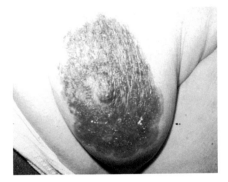

Figure 5.7

A 52-year-old woman presented to the outpatient clinic with an itchy erythematous lesion affecting her left breast.

Questions

Q1 Describe what you see.

Q2 What is the diagnosis? How do you differentiate this from eczema?

Q3 What is the histology of the underlying condition?

Q4 Where else in the body is this condition seen?

Q5 How should this patient be treated?

Answers

(A1) There is an erythematous, eczematous lesion affecting the nipple and areola of the left breast.

(A2) Paget's disease of the nipple.

Table 5.1 Differences between Paget's disease of the nipple and eczema

	Paget's disease	**Eczema**
Cause	Spread of intraductal carcinoma to epidermis	Atopy
Itchy	No	Yes
Bilateral	No	Yes
Vesicular	No	Yes

(A3)
- Paget's disease of the nipple is due to the invasion of the nipple by malignant cells from an underlying tumour.
- Examination can reveal underlying palpable mass (50%) or palpable nodal disease (60%).
- Biopsy will invariably reveal an underlying DCIS or invasive ductal carcinoma.

(A4) The genital region, perineum and axillae.

(A5) Ultimately the patient will require a mastectomy and axillary node dissection. Patients with no obvious mass are likely to have DCIS and should be offered mastectomy or, alternatively, cone excision of the nipple and areola complex, followed by radiotherapy.

Metastatic breast carcinoma

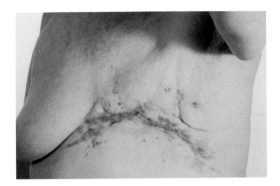

Figure 5.8

Figure 5.8 is taken from a 64-year-old lady who had undergone a previous mastectomy 20 years ago and has now re-presented with a firm nodule in her scar. She was also noted to have dyspnoea and a chest radiograph was also performed (Figure 5.9).

Questions

Q1 What is the most likely diagnosis?

Q2 How is the diagnosis confirmed?

Q3 What is shown on the CXR?

Q4 Apart from the old mastectomy site, where else are you going to examine and investigate?

Q5 What are the principles of treatment of this condition?

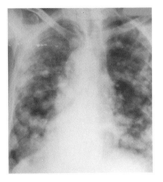

Figure 5.9

Answers

(A1) Local recurrence of the breast cancer. ✔

(A2) Confirm diagnosis with either an FNA or tru-cut biopsy.

(A3) The chest radiograph demonstrates multiple metastases throughout both lung fields.

(A4)
- Examine the back for bony metastases. Check for any evidence of pathological fractures.
- Examine the liver for a hepatomegaly – liver metastases.
- Examine the chest for malignant pleural effusions.
- Check lymph node status – axillary, supraclavicular and sternal chain.
- Check for any evidence of cerebral metastases (CT head scan).
- Check for superior vena cava obstruction.

(A5)
- Systemic chemotherapy for lung metastases. ✔
- Resection for skin ulcerating tumour. ✔
- Pain control with opioids and NSAIDs. ✔
- Internal fixation of long bones for pathological fractures. ✔
- Check for hypercalcaemia: if severe will need correction with intravenous hydration and bisphosphonates.
- Palliative radiotherapy for skeletal metastases and for superior vena cava obstruction secondary to malignant lymphadenopathy. ✔
- Corticosteroids for cerebral metastases. ✔
- Social and psychological support. ✔
- Blood transfusion for anaemia of chronic disease. ✔
- Aspiration of pleural effusions +/− pleurodesis. ✔

Mastectomy and breast reconstruction

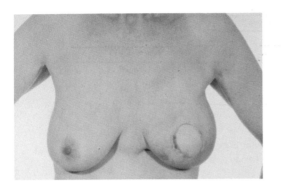

Figure 5.10

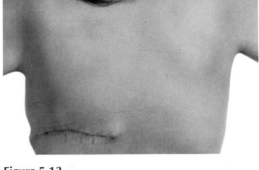

Figure 5.13

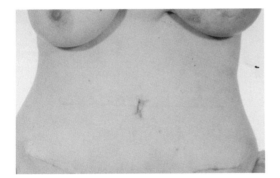

Figure 5.11

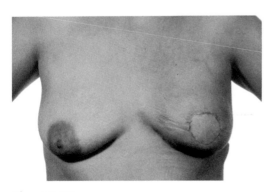

Figure 5.12

Questions

Q1 Look at Figures 5.10 and 5.11. What do they show? Can you link the two?

Q2 What is a mastectomy?

Q3 When would you perform a mastectomy?

Q4 What types of mastectomy do you know about?

Q5 What is breast reconstruction? What are the options?

Q6 Look at Figures 5.12 and 5.13. What type of breast reconstruction has the patient undergone?

Q7 What can be used to reconstruct a breast?

Answers

 • Figure 5.10 shows that there has been surgery on the left breast. There is an ovoid scar over the breast and there is no nipple on that side.
• Figure 5.11 shows a transverse scar across the lower abdomen indicating the donor site of, presumably, a myocutaneous flap reconstruction.
• This patient has had a previous mastectomy probably for carcinoma of the breast with immediate or delayed reconstruction using a transverse rectus abdominis myocutaneous (TRAM) flap.

(A2) Mastectomy is the surgical removal of all breast tissue of one breast.

(A3) **Indications for mastectomy**
• *Therapeutic mastectomy* for carcinoma of the breast:
  – two or more tumours in separate areas of the breast
  – widespread DCIS
  – sub-areola tumour
  – large tumour relative to breast size
  – high risk of further disease (*BRCA1/2* +ve)
  – previous irradiation to the breast
  – when irradiation is contraindicated (e.g. early pregnancy)
  – patient preference.
• *Prophylactic mastectomy*:
  – strong family history of breast carcinoma
  – to obtain optimal symmetry for reconstruction
  – for peace of mind following mastectomy for carcinoma of the contralateral breast.

(A4) **Types of mastectomy**
• *Subcutaneous*: all breast tissue is removed but the overlying skin including the nipple–areola complex remains.
• *Skin-sparing*: all breast tissue and the nipple–areola complex is removed, but the overlying skin remains.
• *Simple* (or total): all breast tissue and overlying skin is removed.
• *Modified radical*: all breast tissue, overlying skin and axillary lymph nodes are removed.
• *Radical*: all breast tissue, overlying skin, pectoralis muscles and axillary lymph nodes are removed. This is very rarely used any more.

 • All women undergoing mastectomy should be offered breast reconstruction, the goal of which is to create a mound to match the remaining natural breast.
• There are three main types of reconstruction – prosthetic, autologous and a combination of the two. Any of these can be performed at the same time as mastectomy (immediate reconstruction) or during a separate operation (delayed reconstruction).
• Immediate reconstruction reduces the psychological trauma of the change in body image experienced after mastectomy, although there is no evidence that it increases the rate of local or systemic relapse. Radiotherapy can be carried out while a prosthesis or expander is *in situ*.
• Delayed reconstruction, although more widely available than immediate surgery, needs a well-healed scar to have formed and generally has poor results following radiotherapy (except in the case of myocutaneous flaps).

Previous mastectomy, presumably for breast carcinoma with immediate or delayed reconstruction using a latissimus dorsi (LD) myocutaneous flap.

- *Prosthetic reconstruction* involves inserting an implant between the chest wall and the pectoralis muscles, which can either be a fixed-volume silicone implant or an expandable saline-filled implant, depending on the nature of the overlying skin and the size of the desired reconstruction. Expanders are then gradually filled with saline over 3–6 months and are then removed and replaced with permanent fixed-volume implants. A relatively recent development is a permanent expandable implant, which has an outer fixed-volume silicone chamber and an inner expandable saline chamber. This allows for tissue expansion and reconstruction in a one-stage procedure.
- *Autologous reconstruction* involves moving tissue from elsewhere to the breast, to create a breast mound. Common donor sites are:
  - the back (LD – muscle and skin)
  - the abdomen (TRAM – muscle, fat and skin; DIEP – fat and skin)
  - the buttock (SGAP/IGAP – fat and skin).
- *Combination reconstruction* is generally used with an LD flap, when the bulk of the muscle itself would not create an adequate mound to match the remaining breast. An implant is inserted between the pectoralis muscles and the transposed latissimus dorsi muscle to increase the volume of the breast while the overlying latissimus dorsi muscle and its skin paddle create a better texture and shape than prosthetic reconstruction alone.

Your revision notes:

Fibroadenoma

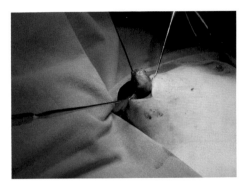

Figure 5.14

This 20-year-old lady is having a discrete lump in her left breast removed. Pre-operative breast ultrasound revealed a well-defined hypo-echoic mass with post-acoustic enhancement.

Questions

Q1 What is the most likely diagnosis? What is the differential diagnosis?

Q2 What are the characteristic clinical features of this mass?

Q3 When does it commonly present?

Q4 Is there a risk of malignancy with this condition?

Q5 What are the treatment options available?

Answers

(A1) These appearances are characteristic of a fibroadenoma. Differential diagnosis of a single discrete lump in the breast is most likely to be:
- fibroadenoma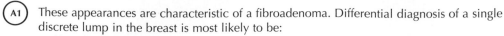
- breast cyst
- breast cancer.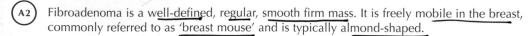

(A2) Fibroadenoma is a well-defined, regular, smooth firm mass. It is freely mobile in the breast, commonly referred to as 'breast mouse' and is typically almond-shaped.

(A3) These are the most common breast lumps in women aged under 35 years (typical age range 15–25 years) but can occur at any age between menarche and menopause. They are hormonally dependent – they increase in size with menstruation and involute after the menopause. Giant fibroadenomas (>5 cm) occur in younger females and are more common in Africa.

(A4) A fibroadenoma is a benign tumour developing from a single breast lobule and is considered an aberration of normal breast tissue development. There is a small risk of malignant change (1/1000) and this is usually an LCIS.

(A5)
- Treatment options are, as always, non-operative and operative.
- Reassure the patient if triple assessment (clinical examination, ultrasound and FNA) confirms diagnosis.
- If the patient is still anxious they can elect to have a lumpectomy as seen in the picture.

Acromegaly

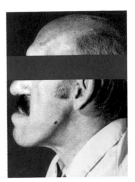

Figure 5.15

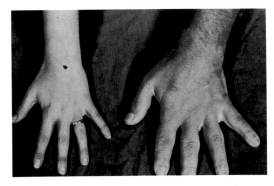

Figure 5.17

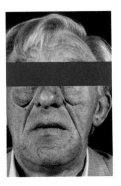

Figure 5.16

Questions

Q1 Look at the three figures. What condition do they depict?

Q2 What clinical features are shown?

Q3 What neurological conditions can this condition cause?

Q4 What are the other associated problems?

Q5 How does this condition come about?

Q6 What are the treatment options?

Q7 Do the signs regress after treatment? What are the signs of active disease?

Answers

(A1) Acromegaly.

(A2) The features shown include:
- thickened greasy skin ✓
- prognathism ✓
- enlarged skull ✓
- prominent lips and nose ✓
- overbite of the lower jaw ✓
- hand enlargement (compared to normal-sized hand). ✓

(A3) Overgrowth of bone and soft tissue can cause:
- carpal tunnel syndrome ✓
- spinal nerve compression giving rise to sciatica ✓
- brachial neuropathy ✓
- optic chiasm compression leading to visual disturbance. ✓

(A4) Associated problems include:
- diabetes ✓
- sleep apnoea ✓
- multinodular goitre ✓
- hypertension ✓
- 2-fold increase in cardiovascular disease ✓
- cardiomyopathy ✓
- left ventricular hypertrophy ✓
- enlarged testes ✓
- increase in malignancies especially colonic polyps ✓
- renal stones (hypercalciuria). ✓

(A5) Acromegaly is almost always due to a GH-secreting tumour. The condition is rarely due to ectopic GH-releasing hormone secretion from a tumour (typically carcinoid), which stimulates the normal pituitary.

(A6)
- First-line treatment is transphenoidal surgery to the pituitary tumour, or transcranial surgery if there is a large suprasellar extension to the tumour. The cure rate depends on the initial tumour size.
- Alternative therapies are octreotide, pituitary radiotherapy or bromocriptine.

(A7)
- Most signs do not regress after treatment.
- Features of active disease are increased sweating and oedema of the hands and feet, which can regress after therapy.

Cushing's syndrome

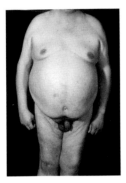

Figure 5.18

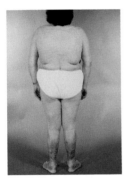

Figure 5.19

A 38-year-old patient presents with a history of recent change in appearance along with weight gain. He also mentioned noticing bruises, which he could not explain. He was found to be hypertensive.

Questions

Q1 What is the likely diagnosis?

Q2 What is the microscopic anatomy of the adrenal gland?

Q3 What are the substances produced by these cells?

Q4 What are the causes of Cushing's syndrome?

Q5 What are the typical clinical features seen in Cushing's syndrome?

Q6 What are the investigations useful in diagnosis and management?

Q7 What are the important aspects of management?

Q8 What are the surgical problems associated with this condition?

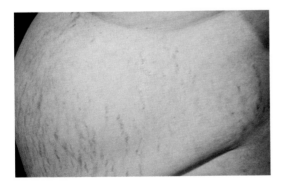

Figure 5.20

Answers

(A1) Cushing's syndrome.

(A2) The adrenal gland consists of a cortex (90%) and medulla (10%) which are developmentally and functionally separate. The cortex consists of three layers: an outer zona glomerulosa, middle zona fasciculata and an inner zona reticularis. The medulla consists of chromaffin cells and preganglionic autonomic nerve fibres from renal and coeliac plexus.

(A3)
- Three classes of corticosteroids are produced by the cortex: mineralocorticoids, glucocorticoids and adrenal androgens.
- The zona glomerulosa produces mineralocorticoids such as aldosterone. Aldosterone acts on the renal distal convoluted tubules to cause sodium reabsorption and excretion of potassium and hydrogen.
- The zona fasciculata and zona reticularis produce glucocorticoids. Cortisol is the main glucocorticoid and has a role in the metabolism of glucose, fat and protein. It increases blood glucose levels.
- The zona fasciculata and zona reticularis also produce androgens. Dehydroepiandrosterone is the main adrenal androgen. It is a weak androgen and the effects only become apparent in adrenal hyperactivity.
- The chromaffin cells of the medulla sythesise, store and secrete catecholamines. Adrenaline, noradrenaline and dopamine are the principal catecholamines. Noradrenaline is the neurotransmitter for the autonomic nervous system. Adrenaline and noradrenaline are present in the adrenals in the ratio of 4:1 and have a half-life of only 1–2 min. Their metabolites metanephrines and VMA are excreted in the urine.

(A4) The causes of Cushing's syndrome are divided into two broad groups:
- *ACTH dependent*: pituitary/hypothalamus-dependent Cushing's disease, ectopic ACTH-secreting tumours and therapeutic excess with ACTH or analogue
- *non-ACTH dependent*: benign and malignant adrenal tumours, macronodular cortical hyperplasia, primary pigmented nodular cortical disease, glucocorticoids or analogues.

(A5) Weight gain, change in body configuration (lemon on sticks appearance), moon facies, skin pigmentation, thin limbs, wasting of muscles, bruising and striae (Figure 5.20), hypertension, osteoporosis, polyuria, impaired glucose tolerance, amenorrhoea, hirsutism, frontal balding, acne, growth retardation, depression, psychosis, venous thrombosis.

(A6) There are three stages of investigations: to confirm hypercortisolism, to determine whether it is ACTH dependent, and imaging to localise the anatomical and pathological abnormality.

Tests to confirm hypercortisolism
- Overnight dexamethasone suppression test: failure to suppress basal levels by 50% or a level >120 nmol/l suggests Cushing's syndrome.
- Urinary free cortisol (normal: 100–350 nmol/24 h).
- Low-level dexamethasone suppression test.

Tests for ACTH dependence
- ACTH assay (normal levels: <25 ng/l at 9 am and <10 ng/l at midnight).
- High-dose dexamethasone suppression test.
- Metyrapone – an enzyme involved in the final stage of cortisol sythesis.
- CRH stimulation of ACTH.
- Bilateral inferior petrosal sinus sampling for ACTH.

Imaging techniques
- Skull imaging to detect microadenomas: CT scan (50% detection), MRI scan (66% detection).
- Adrenals: CT, MRI, isotope scanning (NP59).

- Treatment aims to normalise cortisol levels and return the pituitary and adrenal gland function to physiological control.
- Trans-sphenoidal microadenectomy in Cushing's disease.
- Unilateral adrenalectomy in Cushing's syndrome for an adrenal tumour.
- Bilateral adrenalectomy is no longer the treatment of choice for Cushing's disease. This will lead to lifelong steroid dependence and one-third develop Nelson's syndrome due to an invasive pituitary tumour.

The surgical problems associated with Cushing's syndrome are: poor wound healing, susceptibility to infections, peptic ulcers, fractures, DVT and vascular accidents.

Your revision notes:

Adrenal mass

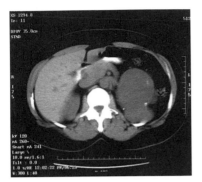

Figure 5.21

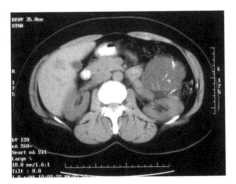

Figure 5.22

This 55-year-old patient had a routine CT scan to investigate long-standing abdominal pain. She has severe, treatment-resistant hypertension.

Questions

Q1 What is the abnormality on the CT scan?

Q2 What are the potential causes of this appearance on CT?

Q3 What is the differential diagnosis in this patient?

Q4 What further simple investigations might be appropriate?

Q5 Would you be more worried about malignancy if she was aged 65 years?

Q6 What are the treatment options for a patient in whom the lesion demonstrated secretion of aldosterone?

Q7 If the management involves surgery, what special precautions need to be taken pre-operatively?

Answers

A1
- Enlarged left adrenal gland.
- The adrenals are 'arrow-like' structures, located superior and anterior to the kidneys in the retroperitoneum.

A2 This question essentially asks what are the causes of an enlarged adrenal gland. Causes can be divided up as usual:

Neoplastic
- *Benign*:
  - adenoma (may be silent or secreting, such as aldosteronoma or Cushing's tumour)
  - paraganglionoma
  - neurofibroma
  - phaeochromocytoma (although 10% are malignant, 10% extra-adrenal, 10% bilateral).
- *Malignant*:
  - adenocarcinoma – rare
  - metastasis (breast, bronchus, melanoma)
  - neuroblastoma (children only).

Cysts
- Usually small and asymptomatic, can cause diagnostic confusion, and they can become large.

Hyperplasia
- Unlikely as this is unilateral.

A3 Essential hypertension is common so any of the above list may be possible, but in a hypertensive individual, the most likely differential diagnoses are the hormone-secreting tumours such as phaeochromocytoma, aldosteronoma (Conn's syndrome) and cortisol-secreting tumour (Cushing's syndrome).

A4 Further investigations will be primarily to investigate the above syndromes:
- urinary catecholamines
- 9 am and midnight serum cortisol
- serum aldosterone and renin (recumbent and ambulant): aldosterone is high in Conn's syndrome, with failure of suppression on ambulation and undetectable plasma renin levels.

A5 No – the risk of malignancy decreases with age.

A6
- A Conn's tumour should be resected if the diagnosis is made confidently (combination of radiology and biochemistry).
- Medical treatment of hypertension with spironolactone, an aldosterone antagonist (see answer to question 7).
- Open versus laparoscopic adrenalectomy:
  - open for large lesions or those with features of malignancy
  - laparoscopic is the standard approach and carries less risk of complications.

- For left adrenalectomy patient is placed lateral and ports placed:
  - transperitoneal approach
  - dissect the lienorenal ligament
  - trace the splenic vein laterally to find the adrenal vein and adrenal gland
  - ligate the veins and remove the adrenal.

- Hypertension and hypokalaemia present anaesthetic risk and both can be addressed by pre-operative therapy with spironolactone. Potassium supplements in refractory cases can be administered.
- Informed consent for laparoscopic adrenalectomy must include open conversion.

Your revision notes:

Phaeochromocytoma

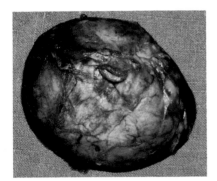

Figure 5.23

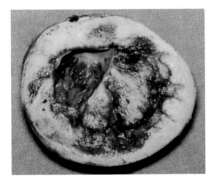

Figure 5.24

A 26-year-old male presented with episodic headache and a sensation of pounding in his chest. His BP was found to be 200/110 mmHg. This mass was subsequently removed from him after investigation.

Questions

Q1 What is the possible cause for his hypertension?

Q2 What are the sites of origin of these tumours?

Q3 What are the clinical features?

Q4 What are the associated conditions?

Q5 How do you confirm the diagnosis?

Q6 What are the important peri-operative measures in its management?

Q7 What are the main principles involved during the surgical operation?

Answers

A1 Phaeochromocytoma.

A2 Phaeochromocytoma is a tumour of chromaffin cells which secrete catecholamines. Most (90%) arise from the adrenal medulla. The remaining 10% arise from extra-adrenal sites such as paraganglionic tissue of the sympathetic chain, and the organ of Zuckercandle. Approximately 10% are bilateral, extra-adrenal, multiple, familial and malignant. Paediatric tumours are more likely (60%) to be malignant.

A3 Hypertension is the principal feature and this is paroxysmal in more than half of the patients. The paroxysms may be brought on by exercise, emotions, Valsalva manoeuvre, drugs and micturition. During the attacks the patient may have chest or abdominal pain and a pounding sensation. They are pale, sweaty and usually tachycardic. MI, pulmonary oedema, hypertensive encephalopathy, stroke, retroperitoneal bleeding, chronic cardiac failure or even sudden death may occur during a pressor crisis. It can also stimulate a diabetic or thyrotoxic state. It is a correctable cause of hypertension and accounts for 1–5 per 1000 new cases of hypertension. The biological actions of the secreted substances dictate the clinical signs. Adrenaline-secreting tumours (adrenal), which stimulate both alpha- and beta-receptors may cause tachycardia and hyperglycaemia. Noradrenaline-secreting tumours (extra-adrenal) activate peripheral $alpha_1$- and $alpha_2$-receptors leading to widespread cutaneous pallor and vasoconstriction. Pressor crisis may be associated with bradycardia.

A4 MEN Type 2 (Sipple syndrome), von Recklinghausen's disease, von Hippel–Lindau disease, Sturge–Weber disease, tuberous sclerosis and acromegaly.

A5 Diagnosis is confirmed by:
- *biochemical tests* to measure catecholamines and their metabolites, e.g. 24-hour urine collection for catecholamines and their metabolites such as VMA, metanephrines, homovanillic acid, 4-hydroxy-3-methoxy mandelic acid
  - normal plasma catecholamine levels: adrenaline, 0.1–0.3 nmol/l and noradrenaline, 0.5–3.0 nmol/l, measured by RIA
- *imaging*: adrenal CT and MRI – adenomas <10 mm can be missed. Venous sampling, MIBG scans (extra-adrenal tumours), 19-iodo-cholesterol (adenoma versus hyperplasia).

A6 Careful control of hypertension is paramount.
- *Pre-operative medications*: initial alpha-blockers (phenoxybenzamine), beta-blockers (propranolol) only after alpha blockade, otherwise a hypertensive crisis can be precipitated. Metirosine is used to suppress catecholamine production.
- *Intra-operative medications*: sodium nitroprusside and phentolamine for hypertension and fluid replacement, dopamine and noradrenaline for hypotension. Handling of the tumour during its excision can result in profound hypertension followed by severe hypotension after its removal.

A7 An open or laparoscopic technique. Both anterior and posterior approaches have been used in open surgery. The important surgical considerations are non-manipulative dissection of the tumour, early control of adrenal vessels, avoidance of capsular rupture, and clearance of adrenal fossa. If there is no appreciable fall in blood pressure after removal, every effort must be made to find multiple tumours.

Parathyroid disease

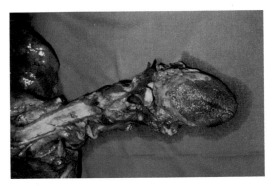

Figure 5.25

Figure 5.25 shows a parathyroid adenoma removed from a patient with primary hyperparathyroidism.

Questions

Q1 What do you know about anatomy and development of the parathyroid gland?

Q2 What do you know about hyperparathyroidism?

Q3 How would you manage primary hyperparathyroidism?

Q4 Are there any investigations that can help locate parathyroid adenoma?

Answers

- There are usually four parathyroid glands. They are intimately related to the posterior border of the thyroid gland. The two superior glands are more constant in position and lie at the level of the middle of the posterior border of thyroid gland, immediately above the termination of the inferior thyroid artery and close to the cricothyroid articulation. The inferior parathyroid glands are more variable in position and can be situated anywhere between the inferior pole of thyroid to the superior mediastinum.
- The superior parathyroid develops from the fourth pharyngeal pouch, and the inferior parathyroid gland from the third pharyngeal pouch. The thymus develops from a diverticulum of the third pharyngeal pouch, and hence it is responsible for the caudal migration of the inferior parathyroid glands.

It is customary to distinguish three categories of hyperparathyroidism:
- *primary hyperparathyroidism*: the most common of the parathyroid disorders. It is characterised by autonomous secretion of PTH usually by a single parathyroid adenoma (90%). Clinical features are related usually to hypercalcaemia. Biochemical abnormalities include elevated calcium and elevated serum PTH.
- *secondary hyperparathyroidism*: this is usually present when there is parathyroid hyperplasia, with PTH secretion in an attempt to compensate for prolonged hypocalcaemia that occurs with chronic renal failure, malabsorption, osteomalacia and rickets. Its effect is to restore serum calcium at the expense of the body skeleton. However, biochemically, the serum calcium is low and PTH is raised.
- *tertiary hyperparathyroidism*: sometimes in a small proportion of cases with secondary hyperparathyroidism, continuous stimulation of the parathyroids may result in adenoma formation and autonomous PTH secretion.

A3 The only corrective treatment is the surgical removal of the overactive gland (adenoma) or glands (hyperplasia). However pre-operative correction of symptomatic hypercalcaemia may be necessary.

A4 The simplest investigation is probably ultrasound examination of the neck. However it is examiner dependent. CT scan is helpful to detect mediastinal parathyroid glands. MRI scan is also used increasingly. Thallium–technetium isotope subtraction imaging may locate 90% of parathyroid adenomas prior to surgery. Technetium (Tc^{99}) and sestamibi can also be used alone due to the differential rate at which they are washed away from the thyroid tissue (10–15 min after injection) and abnormal parathyroid tissue (1.5–3 h after injection).

Index